ECHO

A Vocal Language Program for
Easing Anxiety in Conversation

ECHO

A Vocal Language Program for Easing Anxiety in Conversation

Cesar E. Ruiz, SLPD, CCC-SLP, BCS-S
Evelyn R. Klein, PhD, CCC-SLP, BCS-CL, ASHA Fellow
Louis R. Chesney, BSc

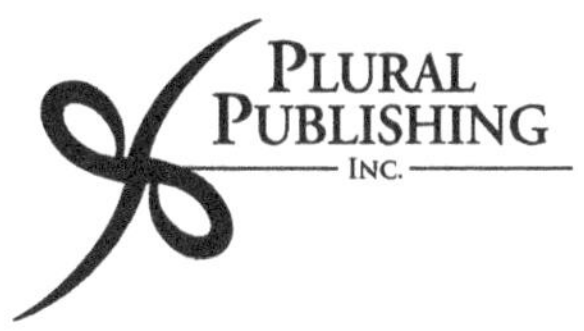

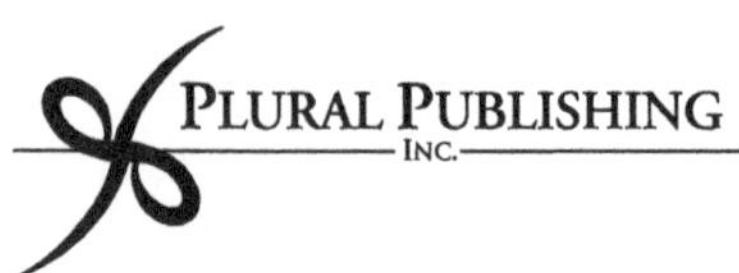

5521 Ruffin Road
San Diego, CA 92123

e-mail: information@pluralpublishing.com
Website: https://www.pluralpublishing.com

Typeset in 11/14 Stone Informal by Flanagan's Publishing Services, Inc.
Printed in the United States of America by Integrated Books International

Library of Congress Cataloging-in-Publication Data

Names: Ruiz, Cesar E. author. | Klein, Evelyn R., author. | Chesney, Louis R., author.
Title: ECHO : a vocal language program for easing anxiety in conversation / Cesar E. Ruiz, Evelyn R. Klein, Louis R. Chesney.
Description: San Diego, CA : Plural Publishing, Inc., [2022] | Includes bibliographical references and index.
Identifiers: LCCN 2021031193 (print) | LCCN 2021031194 (ebook) | ISBN 9781635503302 (paperback) | ISBN 9781635503319 (ebook)
Subjects: MESH: Speech Disorders--therapy | Speech Therapy--methods | Child | Adolescent | Anxiety--therapy | Phobia, Social--therapy
Classification: LCC RC427 (print) | LCC RC427 (ebook) | NLM WL 340.3 | DDC 616.85/506--dc23
LC record available at https://lccn.loc.gov/2021031193
LC ebook record available at https://lccn.loc.gov/2021031194

CONTENTS

ACKNOWLEDGMENTS

We would like to thank the team at Plural Publishing for the opportunity to publish the ECHO Program. The completion of this work would not have been possible without their assistance and the involvement of the individuals acknowledged below. Their contributions have added to the value of this work and are sincerely appreciated and gratefully acknowledged.

We are exceptionally grateful to our contributors, Liz Eckert, MFA, and James Mancinelli, PhD, CCC-SLP. As a cofounder of "Beyond Fluency" and a theater educator, Liz Eckert's work has been invaluable. She has incorporated her experience with improvisation, role-playing, and actor training (including those with disabilities or English as a second language) in the ECHO module on role-play simulations for conversation. We also appreciate the knowledge and clinical experience of Dr. James Mancinelli for his work as a professor and researcher in the field of fluency disorders with specialization in the social aspects of stuttering. His insightful commentaries and clinical suggestions have been incorporated into the ECHO text to support people who stutter.

We are also grateful for the input of Meet Singhal, an engineer by training, and cofounder of Stamurai, for meeting with us and providing insight into the ECHO modules from a person-who-stutters perspective in addition to his own work on program development.

A special thank you is also extended to Katya Pronin for her initial input to the role-play simulations as an educator in the field of applied linguistics. As a cofounder of "Beyond Fluency," she has helped speakers become more expressive.

We thank Rachel Rapp, a former graduate student in the field of communication disorders, for reviewing the ECHO manuscript and online activities, and for providing insightful suggestions about selective mutism from her personal experience.

We would also like to thank our graduate assistants in Communication Sciences and Disorders, Mary Buckley, Taylor Clark, Hannah McKeown, Jacklyn Shragher, and Maureen Stevens, for their help in securing pertinent information for use in this text.

We have been fortunate to work with a very talented editor, Christina Gunning, who was always available to answer our questions and provide expert guidance throughout the writing of this text. We are grateful for the support of Valerie Johns, Executive Editor, and all the talented professionals who work at Plural Publishing for their knowledge and support. In addition, the contributors and reviewers listed are gratefully acknowledged for their expert reviews and suggestions that led to an improved final product.

ABOUT THE CONTRIBUTORS

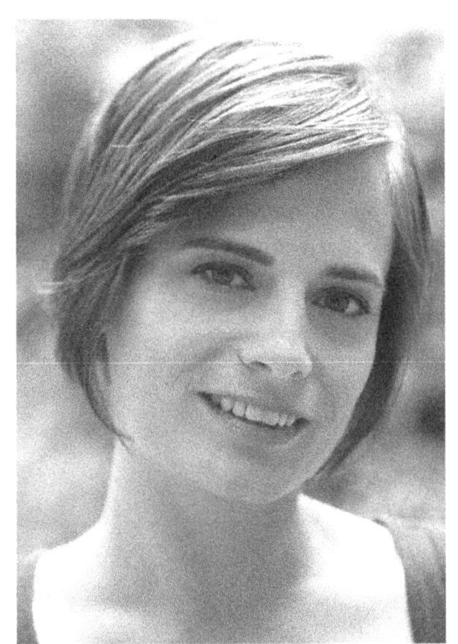

Liz Eckert, MFA, has been a New York–based Designated Linklater Voice Teacher for over 10 years and is currently transitioning her practice to her new home in London. She has held positions on faculties of actor training programs throughout New York City and cofounded Beyond Fluency to help speakers of English as a second language find ease and confidence by engaging with language physically, musically, and sensorially. She has led public speaking workshops at Columbia Business School and conducted role-play training modules with schools and businesses throughout the United States.

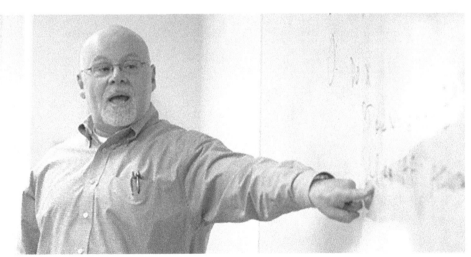

James M. Mancinelli, PhD, CCC-SLP, is an Assistant Professor in the Department of Communication Sciences and Disorders at La Salle University in Philadelphia, Pennsylvania. He has 35 years of clinical experience in medical speech-language pathology and has held senior speech-language pathologist positions at major hospitals in the greater Philadelphia area. He served as the Director of Clinical Education at La Salle University from 2003 to 2019. He teaches the graduate course in Fluency and Stuttering at La Salle University. His research interests include the sociological aspects of stuttering, ethnographic applications to stuttering, conversation analysis as applied to people who stutter, and clinical education/supervision.

REVIEWERS

Plural Publishing and the authors thank the following reviewers for taking the time to provide their valuable feedback during the manuscript development process. Additional anonymous feedback was provided by other expert reviewers.

Kristin Droste, MA, CCC-SLP
Speech-Language Pathologist
Expressions Speech Language and Communication Services, LLC
Garden Grove, California

Joleen R. Fernald, PhD, CCC-SLP, BCS-CL
Speech-Language Pathologist
Joleen R. Fernald Pediatric Therapy Services
Trinity, Florida

Steven Kurtz, PhD, ABPP
Senior Psychologist and President
Kurtz Psychology Consulting PC
New York, New York

Juliana O. Miller, MS, CCC-SLP
Clinical Instructor, Director of External Clinical Practicum
University of South Carolina
Columbia, South Carolina

Robyn M. Newman, PhD, CCC-SLP/L
Speech-Language Pathologist
PediaTalk, LLC
Evanston, Illinois

Rachel Rapp, BA
Graduate Student
Department of Communication Disorders and Sciences
University of Oregon
Eugene, Oregon

Donna Spillman-Kennedy MS, CCC-SLP
Speech-Language Pathologist and Partner
Integrated Speech Pathology, LLC
Watchung, New Jersey

France Weill, PhD, CCC-SLP
Associate Professor
Touro College
New York, New York

INTRODUCTION

The ECHO Program

When choosing a name for this program, we decided on ECHO as an echo involves sound that is produced and reflected back to be heard again. Speech includes a series of sounds that are carefully combined to form words for meaningful language in order to communicate and engage in conversation. Echoes can be heard in such remote places as caves or mountain ranges. This makes an echo a powerful source of sound. We believe that, as humans, we can use communication to achieve meaningful results in our lives.

The ECHO Program was developed for older elementary children and teens who can benefit from social communication experiences to generate voice and ease anxiety with social language skills for conversations and storytelling. This program provides many targeted opportunities to practice through game-like activities and role-play simulations.

Within the ECHO program, there are three targeted modules to expand functional communication in conversation. Module 1 introduces voice initiation techniques and speech sound production from a physiological and mechanical standpoint to make vocalization easier. Module 2 teaches targeted social pragmatic skills to build spontaneous verbal communication for conversation in a hierarchical manner with 11 interactive activities beginning with spontaneity for words and extending to initiating topics during conversation. Module 3 builds on the previous two modules, providing conversational role-plays in simulated settings that incorporate cognitive restructuring. All modules attempt to provide a basis for experiential learning.

Our rationale for serving children and teens with selective mutism or stuttering has to do with the fact that both disorders are impacted by social anxiety related to the demands of speaking. To reduce anxiety, people often avoid situations and that limits their communication experiences over time. Limited experiences speaking can create feelings of discomfort when the person is called upon or expected to engage in speaking tasks that are unfamiliar.

There are many programs available that target social communication and conversation for children and teens. However, none have focused on the impact social anxiety has on voice production and communication, specifically related to selective mutism and stuttering. In our experience as therapists and individuals who have been personally impacted by these disorders, our objective is to offer treatment materials and activities that the therapist or facilitator can readily use to engage and inspire the child or teen to communicate.

Whom the ECHO Program Serves

The ECHO Program was developed for children and teens who have been identified as having selective mutism, childhood-onset fluency disorder (stuttering), and/or have social (pragmatic) communication difficulties. *Selective Mutism* falls within the Anxiety Disorders classification of the *Diagnostic and Statistical Manual of Mental Disorders, Fifth Edition* (*DSM-5*). These disorders are exemplified by excessive fear and anxiety related to behavioral disturbances with anticipation of a future threat. There is a consistent failure to speak in specific social situations in which there is an expectation for speaking such as at school, despite speaking in other situations. *Childhood-Onset Fluency Disorder* falls within the Neurodevelopmental Disorders classification of the *DSM-5*. Normal fluency and time patterning of speech that are inappropriate to the child's age and language skills may be disturbed. Sound and syllable repetitions, prolongations, broken words, blocks, word substitutions, in addition to physical tension are some of the common characteristics. The disturbance causes anxiety about speaking or limitations with effective communication, social participation, or academic or occupational performance. There are persistent difficulties using verbal and nonverbal communication socially for both groups.

According to the American-Speech-Language-Hearing Association (ASHA; https://www.asha.org/Practice-Portal/Clinical-Topics/Selective-Mutism/), while speech-language pathologists are considered appropriate professionals to coordinate the care team for an individual with selective mutism, ASHA urges the

> collaboration between the speech language pathologist (SLP) and behavioral health professionals (such as a school or clinical psychologist, psychiatrist, or school social worker), as well as the classroom teacher and the child's family . . . for appropriate assessment and treatment planning as well as implementation because selective mutism is categorized as an anxiety-based disorder. (Schum, 2002, p. 4)

The same holds true for the information presented on stuttering. Stuttering is a complex, multidimensional disorder for which tension and avoidance are only parts. According to Yaruss, Coleman, and Quesal (2012), "By addressing the child's entire experience of stuttering, clinicians can help children minimize the adverse education and social impact of the disorder while improving children's overall communication success" (p. 542).

Criteria about these disorders from the *DSM-5* are presented in detail in Appendix A (American Psychiatric Association, 2013).

The Modules

Using the ECHO Program, the child or teen is exposed to strategies and situations through 35 face-to-face and interactive activities and games in three modules.

Module 1: Vocal Control

Module 1 introduces voice initiation techniques and speech sound production from a physiological and mechanical standpoint. Oral placement, manner, pitch, and loudness variations are introduced using seven activities for greater ease of vocal initiation and speech production. The activities support individuals with selective mutism and/or stuttering.

Laryngeal/neck tension has been identified in individuals who have selective mutism and those who stutter. The tension and difficulty producing voice have been implicated as a physiological consequence of anxiety. Using surface electromyograph (sEMG), Ruiz and Klein (2018) identified anxiety as a contributor in interfering with the ability to initiate purposeful vocalizations for speech. Their study found that with heightened anxiety there was increased difficulty engaging the vocal system to initiate voice for speech. They found that children with greater laryngeal/neck tension at the level of the thyrohyoid muscle (measured by sEMG) had significantly more laryngeal/neck tension when asked to say their names, prior to initiating any vocalization. This was in contrast to remaining silent, when there was no vocal request. With more time and greater familiarity in the evaluation session, children with selective mutism had significantly decreased levels of anxiety and laryngeal/neck tension. For children and adolescents who stutter, there is increased muscular tension as well. When dysfluencies occur, the individual often recruits muscle groups from surrounding articulatory areas to help overcome blocks. Such behaviors often become classically conditioned and involve recruitment of more muscles that results in the struggle and tension seen in areas of the face, head, and other parts of the body. Irregular breathing, quivering, or tremulous movements may also become evident as stuttering progresses (Ramig & Dodge, 2005). Frustration, pressures, and stigma further exacerbate tension and difficulties for children and teens who stutter or those with selective mutism.

Module 2: Social Pragmatic Communication

This module teaches targeted skills to build spontaneous verbal communication for conversation in a hierarchical manner with 11 interactive activities. This module supports three primary areas of social communication: (1) using language for different reasons, (2) changing language for the listener or situation, and (3) following rules for conversations and storytelling (ASHA, 2020). Within these three categories, interactive and engaging activities build conversational skills with a focus on enhancing communication and reducing anxiety associated with selective mutism, stuttering, and social (pragmatic) communication. Each of the 11 activities include background research and suggestions for modifications when appropriate.

For children who experience selective mutism or stuttering, avoidance is generally a concern. For those with selective mutism, they avoid participating when uncomfortable or remain mute in speaking situations in which they have higher anxiety. For those who stutter, avoidance is also common. Word substitutions may be used when the person who stutters anticipates stuttering on a specific sound or word. There may also be repetitions or prolongations of phonemes or syllables, blocks, pauses, circumlocutions, and physical tension.

This module provides skills to build daily conversations. With the 11 interactive activities and games, the child/teen gains experience to say what comes to mind, expand utterances, engage in and create scripts, follow directions and cope with mistakes, ask and answer yes-no and *wh-* questions, open and close a conversation, keep a conversation going with questions and commenting strategies, stay on topic and move to related topics, share information, tell a story or relate an event, agree and disagree with someone, show appreciation, give compliments, apologize, request clarification, state a problem, make an excuse, make a complaint, and ask for help as well as offer to help someone.

Module 3: Conversational Role-Play Simulations

Module 3 builds on the previous two modules, providing conversational role-plays in simulated real-life settings. Individuals will use their knowledge and training to practice their skills with options for assuming new roles. The conversational role-plays begin with common real-life scenarios based on recollections from people who have had conversational challenges. Photos are used to help imagine the scenarios for the role-plays. Each of the 17 scenarios begins with a story to complete during the role-plays. The individual has the opportunity to finish the story with their own positive, negative, and neutral endings.

The role-play simulations presented in this module correspond to speaking situations in the Selective Mutism Questionnaire (SMQ) (Bergman et al., 2008). The role-play simulations include two different scenarios and interpretations for cognitive reconceptualization from which children and teens can learn new coping skills based on cognitive behavioral therapy. The following cognitive distortions are represented within the 17 scenarios. They include: dichotomous thinking, fortune-telling, catastrophizing, discounting the positive, emotional reasoning, labeling, magnification, minimization, selective abstraction, mind reading, overgeneralization, personalization, should statements, jumping to conclusions, blaming, what if, and unfair comparisons (Kaplan et al., 2017).

The *Cognitive Distortions Questionnaire* (de Oliveira, 2015) was used to help provide information specific to social anxiety (*CD-Quest*). This measure was developed to identify an individual's errors in thinking, consequent emotional states, and maladaptive behaviors (Lang et al., 2016) and formed the framework for the section on cognitive distortions in Module 3. This questionnaire helps measure success for behavioral training and contingency management.

How to Initiate the ECHO Program

Through our clinical experiences as authors and practitioners engaged in therapy with ECHO treatment, we have the following recommendations:

- When meeting the child or teen for the first time, include the parent or someone with whom they feel comfortable. During this time, it is helpful to discuss the treatment and approach you will take.
- The child or teen should agree and want to be part of the treatment process. For older children and teens, they may or may not want their parent to be included during the sessions. With time, it is a good idea for the parent or guardian to leave the sessions, at least partially, to provide time for the child or teen to gain comfort by themself with the facilitator or clinician in a one-on-one or small group setting.
- The communication partner should gather information using the *Information About Me* questionnaire (Appendix C) to learn more about the child or teen. This helps build rapport.
- The sessions should be captivating, using the high-interest activities that are provided. The ECHO activities are available in both print and online versions.
- The facilitator should be perceptive toward the individual's tolerance for environmental stressors. Reduce eye contact and sit next to the child/teen (if in person) instead of across the table. Keep focus on the materials instead of directly on the individual's face. Glancing is a good initial alternative to direct eye contact. See the hierarchy presented in Module 1 for structuring online sessions that systematically introduce exposures from limited visual and verbal interactions to full visual and verbal interactions.
- It is never a good idea to trick or coerce the child or teen to speak or take videos without permission. Some children will allow a video to be made and shared with others, but that cannot be taken for granted and doing so can compromise future interactions.

- Once the child or teen speaks (selective mutism) or talks with less tension about fluency (stuttering), do not make a fuss or show excitement. You can provide labeled praise (saying something positive about what the child actually did) without being overly animated.
- It is best not to interrupt or attempt to fill in words for an individual who is trying to speak. Let them say what they want to say in the time it takes them to say it. You can let them know you have time to listen. If working on decreasing pauses and hastening spontaneous speech output, a visible timer may be used to increase awareness.

Setup for Face-to-Face and Virtual Online Sessions

If working in a private outpatient setting, we recommend meeting with the child or teen and a parent or guardian to introduce the program and tell them what you will be doing together prior to administering any checklists or rating scales. We tell them about the three modules and what is included and why. For children or teens with selective mutism, we tell them that we are not expecting them to speak during this first meeting (online for virtual teletherapy or in person), but they can if they want to. After a few days have passed, we ask the parent/guardian to let us know if their child/teen wants to take part in the program. If so, we proceed with gathering information and scheduling. If the child/teen does not want to engage in treatment, we may try again to find out more about why; if they refuse, we let them know that they can change their mind at any time and tell their parent or guardian to contact us. The ECHO Program can also be part of the school-based therapeutic plan.

Gathering Information

Checklists and rating scales are suggested in addition to a formal clinical evaluation to determine a diagnosis, rule out disorders, and provide additional services, if needed. When beginning to gather information about the client, the following are suggested depending on needs:

1. *The ECHO Checklist* helps the child or teen and facilitator learn about communication skills they believe they have and/or need (Appendix B).
2. The *Information About Me* form helps the facilitator learn more about the interests, hobbies, activities, and things the individual likes to do. The child/teen can complete it in writing and/or through interview (Appendix C).
3. The *Social Communication Skills—The Pragmatics Checklist* (Goberis et al., 2012), also in Module 2 of this book, provides an array of social pragmatic skills for the child or teen to rate themselves and to learn more about how much they communicate using 45 social communication skills (Appendix D).
4. The *Selective Mutism Questionnaire* (Bergman et al., 2008) is a norm-referenced measure with 17 items that are rated for speaking frequency in school, at home, and in social situations outside school. The measure can be accessed at the following link: https://www.oxfordclinicalpsych.com/view/10.1093/med:psych/9780195391527.001.0001/med-9780195391527-interactive-pdf-002.pdf
5. An online *Case History Form* (Super Duper, 2004) is provided to gather important information about the individual's background. The form can be accessed at the following link: https://www.superduperinc.com/caseHistory/caseHistory.pdf

6. The *EXPRESS Selective Mutism (SM) Communication Questionnaire* (Klein et al., 2018) provides background information with a matrix for rating whom the child or teen speaks to, where, and how (Appendix E).
7. The *Screen for Child Anxiety Related Disorders (SCARED) Questionnaire* (Birmaher et al., 1999) has both child and parent versions for rating characteristics of related anxiety disorders that may be ruled out or require referral for additional support. The measure can be accessed at the following link: https://www.midss.org/content/screen-child-anxiety-related-disorders-scared (Scroll to the bottom of the main page for parent and child scoring forms.)
8. A *Stuttering Attitudes Checklist* can provide useful information about the individuals and thoughts about stuttering in their life. The checklist can be accessed at the following link: http://trittspeech-language.pbworks.com/f/fluency.pdf
9. The *Person-Centered Focus on Function for School-age Children* incorporates the International Classification of Functioning, Disability, and Health model with guidance from the ASHA about stuttering. See the information at the following link: https://www.asha.org/siteassets/uploadedFiles/ICF-School-Age-Stuttering.pdf
10. The CALMS Rating Scale provides measurement guidelines for cognitive, affective, linguistic, motor, and social ratings related to stuttering (Kaufman, 2005). See the rating scale at the following link: https://hhs.uncg.edu/csd/wp-content/uploads/sites/1009/2020/06/2.D.._CALMS_rating_form1.pdf

Connections Between Social Anxiety and Communication

Social anxiety is a concomitant concern for children and teens with selective mutism and/or stuttering. Social anxiety can negatively impact communication, disrupting working memory that is needed to attend to and process what someone else says and respond or initiate with ease (Moran, 2016). Individuals experiencing social anxiety feel uncertain about what to say and over time lack practice speaking and conversing. Their fearfulness takes up much needed working memory capacity. With increased concern or worry about speaking, individuals attempt to reduce their level of anxiety by avoiding people and places.

Stuttering and selective mutism can be concomitant disorders. Speech and language difficulties are known to be risk factors for developing stuttering (Seery et al., 2007) as well as selective mutism (Sharp et al., 2007). Both have a relationship to social anxiety and fear of negative evaluation (Iverach, Menzies, et al., 2011). According to K. Scaler Scott (2018), negative reactions related to stuttering have been known to manifest in outward symptoms of selective mutism.

The anxiety-based thought process for people experiencing selective mutism or stuttering may be experienced according to Clark and Wells (1995) and Rapee and Heimberg (1997). Following are thoughts that may be anticipated by an older child or teen who encounters a social situation in which they are expected to speak:

- There is an anticipation of a social situation that will incite fear *(Everyone will hear me).*
- Then negative thoughts and beliefs arise about oneself in the social situation *(I am no good in social situations, I have trouble talking).*

- The individuals then extend their attentional biases and self-focus on external cues *(People will be looking at me and think poorly of me)* and internal cues *(I will blush, my heart will beat fast, I'll be lightheaded, I'll feel like I am choking).*
- Next, strategies and safety behaviors such as avoidance rush in to reduce the anxiety and discomfort *(I will try to rehearse what I need to say, I'll avoid eye contact, I won't say certain words, I won't speak, I'll escape).*
- After the event, there are post-event thoughts and processing that take place *(I couldn't get my words out, I failed)*, which leads back to negative thoughts and beliefs about oneself in the situation and consequent self-focus, which once again repeats the cycle of avoidance for eye contact, words, and situations or other safety behaviors such as mental rehearsal, using safe words, staying with selected people, or escaping. This leads to feelings of defeat in situations where the individual is expected to speak socially (Iverach, Rapee, et al., 2017, p. 543).

Koç and Dündar (2018) investigated social anxiety and communication skills in 382 school students. They found that students with poorer communication skills (measured with the Communication Skills Scale; Korkut, 1997) had significantly higher levels of social anxiety ($p = .003$) as measured by the Social Anxiety Scale (Ozbay & Palanci, 2001). Those with higher social avoidance scores had lower basic communication skills and experienced greater feelings of worthlessness and overall social anxiety. As basic communication skills increased, social avoidance, anxiety, and feelings of worthlessness decreased. As self-expression increased, social avoidance, evaluation anxiety, feelings of worthlessness, and social anxiety also decreased. There was an inverse relationship with social anxiety and communication skills. With reduced experiences talking to a variety of people in various situations, speaking becomes less comfortable and more challenging.

Halls, Cooper, and Creswell (2015) investigated communication deficits and social anxiety disorder. Parents completed the Social Communication Questionnaire (SCQ) (Rutter et al., 2003) about their children. A total of 262 children had a diagnosis of social anxiety disorder, and 142 were identified as being anxious but without a diagnosis of social anxiety disorder. The children with social anxiety disorder scored significantly higher on all domains of the SCQ (i.e., poor social interaction, communication difficulties, and repetitive, restrictive behaviors) indicating more impairment than the children with nonsocial forms of anxiety. The authors concluded that social communication skills are important in treating social anxiety disorder. Rapee and Spence (2004) also believe that communication deficits may underlie social anxiety disorder and suggest that those with social communication difficulties receive treatment to improve social skills and reduce avoidance in social situations.

In a study by Klein, Ruiz, Morales, and Stanley (2019), parents of 38 children diagnosed with selective mutism rated their children using the Behavior Assessment System for Children, Third Edition (BASC-3). Parents identified *Withdrawal* as "clinically significant" and *Social Skills* and *Functional Communication* as "at-risk" in their children. Teachers rated the same group of children. Those with better social skills scored statistically, significantly higher on standardized and norm-referenced measures of vocabulary, narrative language comprehension, and auditory serial memory (Peabody Picture Vocabulary Test-4, Test of Narrative Language-2, and Test of Auditory Processing Skills-3, respectively).

Gary Renschler (2014), in his manual, *A Clinician's Guide to the Stuttering Clinic*, clearly stated that when demands become too overwhelming for the speech system, disruptions of fluency occur, and effortless speech becomes effortful and uncoordinated. Speech also becomes difficult when muscles used for producing voice become tense. The tension generally comes from anxiety, specifically related to potential frustration and embarrassment the individual feels. In response, people who stutter (PWS) may avoid situations or words to help reduce demands on their speech system. By avoiding, they limit their experiences.

According to Renschler (2014), anxiety and fear are central to stuttering. Consequently, beliefs arise that intensify the person's fears and begin to cultivate negative perceptions related to speaking. Negative thinking from past experiences and negative memories further impacts the person's ability to speak with ease. Some people experience a "fight-or-flight" sensation that makes communication nearly impossible. When this happens, respiration is usually affected, and higher-order thinking becomes challenged. Some people who stutter would rather not speak than stutter. Renschler believed that anxiety and fearfulness could be a bigger problem than stuttering itself. When a person is in a state of heightened anxiety, they can have trouble thinking and experience a rapid heart rate, perspiration, dry mouth, headache, stomachaches, and other physiological symptoms. This negatively impacts communication.

Adolescents who stutter have an increased rate of social anxiety (Gunn et al., 2014). Iverach, Rapee, Wong, and Lowe (2017) support the notion that social anxiety in stuttering is maintained by fear of negative social evaluation and cognitions, use of safety behaviors, self-focus, and anticipatory and postevent processing. Research with a large sample of school-age children who sought treatment for stuttering found that 24% also met criteria for a diagnosis of social anxiety disorder (Iverach, Jones, et al., 2016). The percentages increase with age. According to Blumgart, Tran, and Craig (2010), between 22% and 66% of adults who stutter have been diagnosed with a comorbid anxiety disorder. Anxiety with anticipation of an oncoming speech struggle can make a person who stutters worry about being criticized. With anxiety, the person who stutters may want to avoid responding, and that impacts their conversational experiences.

Dysfluencies have been associated with both stuttering and selective mutism (Scott, 2018). Difficulties engaging in social language can lead to hesitations, reformulations, use of frequent filler words, and intermittent dysfluencies in children who stutter as well as children with selective mutism. According to Weiss (2004), pragmatic language intervention has been found to support children who stutter.

The ARC Model—Generalizing Skills

The ARC (*Anxiety Tolerance, Rescue Reduction,* and *Communication Confidence*) Model (Klein et al., 2021) is presented to gain a better understanding of anxiety as it impacts communication. The model provides information that can be shared with parents or guardians to help them gain a greater understanding of the anxiety-rescue-communication cycle. With this information comes awareness of a conceptual change that may seem counterintuitive at first but should help move the child or adolescent from safety-seeking behaviors to greater confidence communicating.

The ARC Model (Figure 0–1) was developed to help the facilitator of the ECHO Program integrate three characteristics of anxiety, specifically related to children and teens who experience anxiety and social communication deficits. Figure 0–1 provides a visual image of the model, moving from safety-seeking behaviors toward confidence that supports functional communication. The goal is to move up the hill from reliance on safety behaviors that limit communication

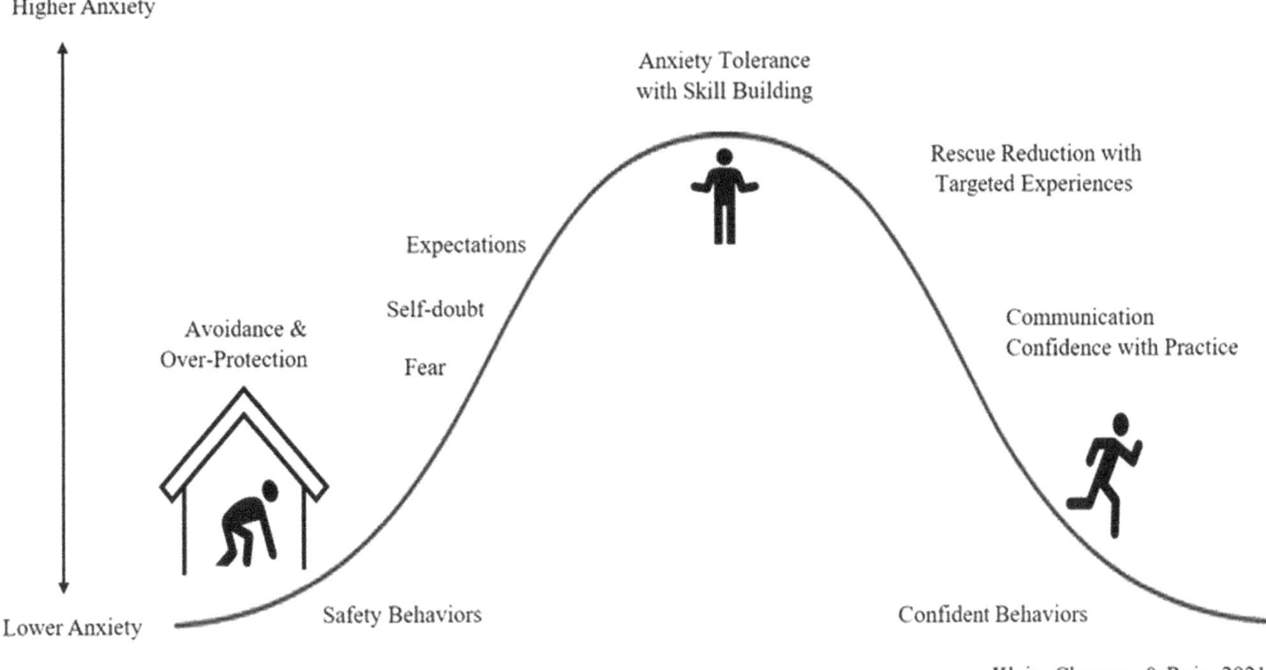

FIGURE 0–1. ARC Model for anxiety tolerance, rescue reduction, and communication confidence.

experiences and progress down the other side toward feelings of confidence during communication experiences. Progression generally occurs in the following manner.

Anxiety Tolerance

Anxiety tolerance can be beneficial in reducing the need for safety behaviors. Safety behaviors are actions people take when feeling anxious to reduce their discomfort, uneasiness, or worry. Avoidance and escape are common safety behaviors and may include not talking or staying away from places or people where there is an expectation to speak. However, this does not help the person eliminate anxiety related to expectations, self-doubt, and fear in the long term. In fact, it does the opposite, and with greater avoidance comes less interactions and less opportunities. By not avoiding but tolerating anxiety in stages, it becomes minimized, desensitized, and ultimately extinguished. This requires *anxiety tolerance*.

Rescue Reduction

Rescue reduction is a process that reduces negative reinforcement. Negative reinforcement is a powerful contributor in keeping a behavior going. The person who continues to rescue the child or teen by speaking for them or accepting avoidance is enabling the problem in some way. The rescuer is usually unaware of the effects. In fact, they think they are helping the person. To combat learned avoidance, individuals cannot run away from their difficulties, they must address them.

Communication Confidence

The ultimate goal within the ARC Model is *communication confidence.* We want to help the child or teen cope with not being rescued unnecessarily, and we want to guide and support them to participate in the many joys that come from interacting and communicating with others at school, in public social settings, as well as at home when people other than the immediate family visit. Even when the child or teen refuses to attempt a skill or states they cannot do a specific task, they need to know it can be modified and made easier for them or tried later when they feel more capable. Encourage them to think about things that were once difficult but that they learned to do. Riding a bike, learning to read, and using a computer or cell phone are just a few common examples. Help the child or teen change their mental imagery of themselves. This has been found to reduce social anxiety during conversations (Leigh et al., 2020).

Some characteristics that reduce social anxiety and make an individual a more comfortable communication partner include an easygoing nature, being non-judgmental, non-critical, non-intimidating, non-pressuring, not overly enthusiastic, and presenting as a calm, humble, and supportive person.

Documentation and Progress

Parents of children with whom the authors have worked noted, *"Your program has given a tremendous boost to our child's progress, beyond anything that we have seen in prior therapies!"* When asked to rate sessions on a scale of 1 (not very helpful) to 5 (very helpful), a teenage client rated sessions as "6" and indicated that she has a *"fear of being judged"* and that *"the activities are giving me practice and more confidence to speak."* Another client's teacher noted that, *"He is having more of a presence in the class with his peers."* And, another client noted, *"I am improving with my tone of voice and expression when I speak."* As a result of using ECHO, children who have been mute have gained skills in making phone calls to a variety of stores to learn about a product, to recreational establishments for information, and to restaurants for ordering food. They have delivered prepared presentations in front of the class, and spoken to teachers, asking for needed information. They have also greeted others and engaged in conversations with friends. These were children who had not made progress previously with other programs. The vocal control approach was the initial strategy used. We have used the vocal control approach with 42 children and adolescents who have come to the University Community Clinic for speech-language evaluations for selective mutism (Ruiz & Klein, 2018) and did not speak upon entry and in most public encounters of their lives. Approximately 93% of the children were able to initiate their voices with ease by the end of the session. Parents were consistently surprised and elated at what they learned and saw during the initial comprehensive evaluation.

The following information represents average case improvements on the SMQ (Selective Mutism Questionnaire; Bergman et al., 2008).

> Scores on the SMQ range from 0 = *never*; 1 = *seldom*; 2 = *often*; to 3 = *always* and relate to frequency of speaking in 17 situations.

At School	(pre) 1.33/(post) 1.83
With Family	(pre) 1.4/(post) 2.2
In Social Situations	(pre) 0.6/(post) 1.6
Total	(pre) 18/(post) 30 points (out of total 51 possible)

Interpretation of the SMQ indicates substantial improvements.

Additional speaking has extended to teachers and school staff, peers at school, family members who do not live with the child, family members in unfamiliar places, family friends, doctors, waiters, and clerks.

Noted improvements in communicative interactions:

- Reduction in hesitations (extended pauses) from an average of 20 seconds to less than 4 seconds in response to saying an associated word.
- Responses to questions increased from answering with one word to using complete sentences.
- (Child's name) learned to make comments to others' statements and ask *wh-* questions in response to someone else speaking.
- (Child's name) sentence completion responses improved to include the following:
  - □ "When I share information with someone, *I try to make them understand what I say.*"
  - □ "When someone else is talking, *I listen to them and respond.*"
  - □ "When speaking with someone, *I want to have a good conversation with them.*"
  - □ And they are spontaneously expanding answers to questions beyond the single word responses previously given.

Comments from parents:

- "I was so surprised and thrilled that (child's name) was able to tell the waiter what she wanted for dinner! That was just wonderful, and she even was answering my questions when we were out on the parking lot."
- A grandparent, who reported after engaging in dialogue with her teenage granddaughter for the first time, told parents of the child, "You must be so happy with her progress!"
- "The role-playing is surely good practice for (child's name). In terms of results, at the competition last week, (child's name) engaged with another child and said, 'I did a good job.'"
- "Last week (child's name) went with a group of friends to a farm for a hayride. She was not inhibited in front of other parents! Afterward we went for ice cream. We were in line and she asked for money since a few friends were buying on their own and she wanted to do the same. . . . After a few seconds, she said 'chocolate' for the flavor."
- "(Child's name) told us that she asked her teacher a question in school and that was the first time she has ever done that."
- "[For a class project,] she did a rap song as a project in front of class with another student."

- Toward the completion of the ECHO Program, a client who attended an orientation at a new high school, spontaneously gave their name and said what they were interested in studying for the future, in front of the group.
- "Our child has been seen by some of the biggest names in the field over the past 6 years. Using this program, it is the best result we have had to date!"

Comments from teachers:

- "(Child's name) did a great job today. (Child's name) came right up and the two got started [speaking in front of the class for their debate project.] After the other child presented her perspective, (child's name) looked at her and asked three questions she had practiced. When it was (child's name) turn to present her perspective, she did a great job. She began to read aloud, and [other students] said that others could hear her loud and clear in the back of the room. As she was reading, she would look up at the audience here and there as she was presenting her piece."

References

American Psychiatric Association. (2013). *Diagnostic and statistical manual of mental disorders* (5th ed.).

American Speech-Language-Hearing Association. (2020). *Person-centered focus on function for school-age children.* https://www.asha.org/siteassets/uploadedFiles/ICF-School-Age-Stuttering.pdf

Bergman, R. L., Keller, M. L., Piancentini, J., & Bergman, A. J. (2008). The development and psychometric properties of the selective mutism questionnaire. *Journal of Clinical Child and Adolescent Psychology, 37*(2), 456–464. https://doi.org/10.1080/15374410801955805

Birmaher, B., Brent, D. A., Chiappetta, L., Bridge, J., Monga, S., & Baugher, M. (1999). Psychometric properties of the Screen for Child Anxiety Related Emotional Disorders (SCARED): A replication study. *Journal of the American Academy of Child and Adolescent Psychiatry, 38*(10), 1230–1236.

Blumgart, E., Tran, Y., & Craig, A. (2010). Social anxiety disorder in adults who stutter. *Depression and Anxiety, 27*, 687–692.

Clark, D. M., & Wells, A. (1995). The cognitive model of social phobia. In R. G. Heimberg, M. R. Liebowitz, D. A. Hope, & F. R. Schneier (Eds.), *Social phobia: Diagnosis, assessment and treatment* (pp. 69–93).

de Oliveira, I. R. (2015). Introducing the Cognitive Distortions Questionnaire. In I. R. de Oliveira (Ed.), *Trial-based cognitive therapy: A manual for clinicians* (pp. 25–40). Routledge.

Goberis, D., Beams, D., Dalpes, M., Abrisch, A., Baca, R., & Yoshinaga-Itano, C. (2012). The missing link in language development: Social communication development. *Seminars in Speech and Language, 33*(4), 297–309.

Gunn, A., Mexzies, R. G., O'Brian, S., Onslow, M., Packman, A., Lowe, R., . . . Block, S. (2014). Axis I anxiety and mental health disorders among stuttering adolescents. *Journal of Fluency Disorders, 40*, 58–88.

Halls, G., Cooper, P. J., & Creswell, C. (2015). Social communication deficits: Specific associations with social anxiety disorder. *Journal of Affective Disorders, 172*, 1, 38–42. https://doi.org/10/1016/j.jad.2014.09.040

Iverach, L., Jones, M., McLellan, L. F., Lyneham, H. J., Menzies, R. G., Onslow, M., & Rapee, R. M. (2016). Prevalence of anxiety disorders among children who stutter. *Journal of Fluency Disorders, 49*, 13–28.

Iverach, L., Menzies, R. G., O'Brian, S., Packman, A., & Onslow, M. (2011). Anxiety and stuttering: Continuing to explore a complex relationship. *American Journal of Speech-Language Pathology, 20*(3), 221–232.

Iverach, L., Rapee, R. M., Wong, Q. J. J., & Lowe. R. (2017). Maintenance of social anxiety in stuttering: A cognitive-behavioral model. *American Journal of Speech-Language Pathology, 26*, 540–556.

Kaplan, S. C., Morrison, A. S., Goldin, P. R., Olino, T. M., Heimberg, R. G., & Gross, J. J. (2017). The cognitive distortions questionnaire (CD Quest): Validation in a sample of adults with social anxiety disorder. *Cognitive Therapy Research, 41*, 576–587.

Kaufman, E. (2005 October 22). *Using the Calms model as a thematic approach to fluency therapy*. Louisiana State University at Baton Rouge. https://www.mnsu.edu/comdis/isad8/papers/kaufman8.html

Klein, E. R., Armstrong, S. L., Gordon, J., Kennedy, D. S., Satko, C. G., & Shipon-Blum, E. (2018). *EXPRESS: Expanding receptive and expressive skills through stories*. Plural Publishing.

Klein, E. R., Chesney, L., & Ruiz, C. E. (2021). *The ARC model* [Lecture notes]. Department of Communication Sciences and Disorders, La Salle University.

Klein, E. R., Ruiz, C. E., Morales, K., & Stanley, P. (2019). Variations in parent and teacher ratings of internalizing, externalizing, adaptive skills, and behavioral symptoms in children with selective mutism. *International Journal of Environmental Research and Public Health, 16*(21), 4070. https://doi.org/10.3390/ijerph16214070

Koç, M., & Dündar, A. (2018). Research on social anxiety level and communication skills of secondary school students. *Asian Journal of Education and Training, 4*(4), 257–265. https://doi.org/10.20448/journal.522.2018.44.257.265

Korkut, F. (1997). Evaluating communication skills of university students. *National Educational Sciences Congress 4th* (pp. 208–218). Anadolu University, Eskisehir.

Lang, C., Nir, Z., Gothelf, A., Domachevsky, S., Ginton, L., Kushnir, J., & Gothelf, D. (2016). The outcome of children with selective mutism following cognitive behavioral intervention: A follow-up study. *European Journal of Pediatrics, 175*, 481–487. https://doi.org/10.1007/s00431-015-2651-0

Leigh, E., Chiu, K., & Clark, D. M. (2020). The effects of modifying mental imagery in adolescent social anxiety. *PLOS ONE, 15*(4), e0230826. https://doi.org/10.1371/journal.pone.0230826

Moran, T. P. (2016). Anxiety and working memory capacity: A meta-analysis and narrative review. *Psychological Bulletin, 142*, 831–864. https://doi.org/10.1037/bul0000051

Ozbay, Y., & Palanci, M. (2001). *Social anxiety scale: Validity, reliability study*. VI. National Psychological Counseling and Guidance Congress. Ankara, ODTÜ.

Ramig, P. R., & Dodge, D. M. (2005). *The child and adolescent stuttering treatment and activity resource guide*. Thomson Delmar Learning.

Rapee, R. M., & Heimberg, R. G. (1997). A cognitive-behavioral model of anxiety in social phobia. *Behavior Research and Therapy, 35*, 741–756.

Rapee, R. M., & Spence, S. H. (2004). The etiology of social phobia: Empirical evidence and an initial model. *Clinical Psychological Review, 24*, 737–767.

Renschler, G. J. (2014). *Clinician's guide to the stuttering clinic*. http://www.mnsu.edu/comdis/kuster/teaching/rentschler/Rentschler-StutteringClinicManual.html

Ruiz, C. E., & Klein, E. K. (2018). Surface electromyograph to identify laryngeal tension in selective mutism: Could this be the missing link? *Biomedical Journal of Scientific & Technical Research, 12*(2), 1–4. https://doi.org/10.26717/BJSTR.2018.12.002222

Rutter, M., Bailey, A., & Lord, C. (2003). *The social communication questionnaire*. Western Psychological Services.

Schum, R. (2002). Selective mutism: An integrated approach. *The ASHA Leader, 7*(17), 4–6. https://doi.org/10.1044/leader.FTR1.07172002.4

Scott, K. S. (2018). *Fluency plus: Managing fluency disorder in individuals with multiple diagnoses*. Slack.

Seery, C. H., Watkins, R. V., Mangelsdorf, S. C., & Shigeto, A. (2007). Subtyping stuttering II: Contributions form language and temperament. *Journal of Fluency Disorders, 32*(3), 197–217.

Sharp, W. G., Sherman, C., & Gross, A. M. (2007). Selective mutism and anxiety: A review of the current conceptualization of the disorder. *Journal of Anxiety Disorders, 21*(4), 568–579.

Super Duper Publications. (2004). *Speech-language-hearing case history form*. https://www.superduperinc.com/caseHistory/caseHistory.pdf

Weiss, A. L. (2004). Why we should consider pragmatics when planning treatment for children who stutter. *Language, Speech, and Hearing Services in Schools, 35*, 34–45.

Yaruss, J. S., Coleman, C. E., & Quesal, R. W. (2012). Stuttering in school-age children: A comprehensive approach to treatment. *Language Speech Hearing Service School, 43*(4), 536–548. https://doi.org/10.1044/0161-1461(2012/11-0044)

Module 1

VOCAL CONTROL: GAINING CONTROL OF YOUR VOICE FOR SPEECH INITIATION

Background Introduction and Theoretical Framework

Voice production starts at the time we are born. Our cry signifies the beginning of life as well as a future communication tool. Voice initially manifests itself in a spontaneous manner and gradually develops into speech sounds. Voice production, however, is a complex process that requires the coordination of several systems (Bouchard et al., 2013; Davis et al., 1996; Jürgens, 2009).

The activities are presented in a hierarchical format with goals to teach how speech sounds are made and to improve purposeful voice initiation and control to express wants and needs. This module is valuable even if one can make speech sounds with ease. As children/teens engage in these activities, the mystery about how we talk is reduced. This helps them feel less anxious and more at ease about speaking. Children/teens learn how to manipulate their voice, modify loudness and pitch, produce speech on demand, and use intonation to identify and convey emotions. Each activity in this module contains the goals of the activity, materials, and how to play. The seven activity titles follow in italics:

1. *Sound Off:* Speech sound production
   - Airflow (continuous or stop)
   - Variations in mouth, nose, and throat sounds (feeling vibration and placement)
2. *Pitch Pipe:* Changing pitch
   - Voice pitch activities (high, normal, low)
3. *Ramp It Up:* Changing loudness
   - Voice loudness activities (loud, normal, soft, whisper)
4. *Vocal Marathon:* Freeing the voice
   - Learning to control and release vocal tension purposefully
5. *Tag Along:* Generation of new words
   - Increasing awareness of sound placement, manner, and voicing (coarticulation)
6. *What's Up?* Answering questions
   - Using vocal control to answer direct questions (who, what, where, when, why, and how)

7. *Let's Face It:* Emotions with voice
   - Using voice to convey emotions (happy, sad, angry, anxious, and disgusted)

Proposed Hierarchy for Face-to-Face and Online Sessions: How to Begin

For in-person face-to-face work, the parent/guardian may be present for some or all of the initial session to facilitate communication as needed. Table 1–1 provides some guidance on how sessions may need to be structured. (This information is based on the authors' professional clinical experiences.)

Children/teens with Selective Mutism often need support when beginning therapy with someone new. Therefore, an extra table has been added with specific modifications to the heirarchy for teletherapy. Depending on the age of the child, we advise that the parent or guardian be part of the first session. We also advise that the facilitator be able to modify audio and video components when using teletherapy format. For in-person face-to-face work, the parent/guardian may be present for some or all of the initial session to facilitate communication as needed. Table 1–2 provides guidance on how sessions with children with selective mutism may need to be structured. The proposed charts may be modified as needed.

In working with children/teens who stutter, we encourage comfort with stuttering and spontaneous fluency (Sisskin, 2018). Using a multifactorial model, dysfluent speech incorporated a

TABLE 1–1. Hierarchy for Face-to-Face Sessions for Selective Mutism

Step 1	Introduction session with parent and child/teen—Facilitator provides information about self and the program and what they will be doing together related to the work within the modules. Child/teen may speak directly or through parents.*
Step 2	Parent is present initially. The facilitator begins discussing how sound production and voicing take place. It is best if the child/teen tolerates their voice to be heard by the facilitator as they speak to the parent. Responses from child/teen may also include pointing, nodding, circling or underlining responses, or drawing, as communication is the primary intention.
Step 3	Parents may be involved to help with activities. Facilitator may avert eye contact and use defocused communication at times (so attention is not always on the child/teen). Responses from child/teen are verbal (reading aloud, simple phrases, and responding). Audible whispers (whispers that can be heard) are acceptable as this reduces vocal fold tension.
Step 4	Parents close by, if needed. Child/teen responses are verbal, may face away or use a barrier between facilitator and child/teen. *Open-ended* (*wh-*) questions may change to *choice* questions (giving two or three options) and then to *yes/no* questions, depending on responses. Child/teen may record their response on a recording device, away from the facilitator, and return to play it. Audible whispers are acceptable as this reduces vocal fold tension.
Step 5	Parents may or may not be close by. Child/teen responds with words, phrases, sentences, and spontaneous verbal output. *Open-ended* (*wh-*) questions may change to *choice* questions (giving two or three options) and then to *yes/no* questions, depending on responses. Voice may be quiet but audible, not a whisper.
Step 6	Child/teen responds and initiates using words, phrases, sentences, and spontaneous verbal output. Voice is audible.

Note: *Parents or guardian or sibling or selected friend may be part of the follow-up sessions, as determined.

dynamic pathways theory (Smith & Weber, 2017). Overtime stuttering is impacted by the struggle to maintain fluency compounded by tension, embarrassment, and feeling of lack of control. Using the Avoidance Reduction Therapy for Stuttering (ARTS) approach by Vivian Sisskin (2018), the goal is to reduce avoidance reactivity and detrimental thinking that often leads to greater struggle. Responses from child/teen include reduction of effort to control or manage one's stuttering. This is a framework that we want to incorporate within the ECHO Program (Table 1–3).

TABLE 1–2. Heirarchy for Online Sessions for Children/Teens With Selective Mutism

Step 1	For this part, the facilitator will be speaking primarily to the parent so the video and sound are best to be on. At this point, the child/teen can remain silent, use the chat tool or speak through parents or directly to the facilitator.
Step 2	The child/teen may want to leave the video and sound off initially. They may use the chat feature to communicate with the facilitator.
Step 3	Parents close by. Leave the video on and turn the audio off. Responses from child/teen may be with gestures and online *chat* feature to communicate in writing.
Step 4	Parents close by, if needed. Video *on* and sound *off*, but to come *on* for responses. Child/teen may turn away from view if needed.
Step 5	Parents close by, if needed. Video and sound remain *on* for the duration of the session. Child/teen may turn away from the camera, but responses are to be verbal.
Step 6	Parents close by, if needed. Video and sound remain *on* for the duration of the session. Child/teen should face the camera, and responses are to be verbal.

Note: Parents or guardian or sibling or selected friend may be part of the follow-up sessions, as determined.

TABLE 1–3. Hierarchy for Face-to-Face and Online Sessions for Children/Teens Who Stutter

Step 1	Introduction session with parent and child/teen—Facilitator to provide information about self and the program and what they will be doing together related to the work within the modules.
Step 2	*Parent may be present initially. Orientation to sound production and voicing. It is best if the child/teen exhibits less reactivity related to stuttering and at the same time does not suppress dysfluencies. If online, video may be off initially, if desired.
Step 3	Facilitator may avert eye contact and use defocused communication at times (so attention is not always on the child/teen). Responses from child/teen are verbal (reading aloud, simple phrases, and responding). The child/teen focuses on the task rather than trying to maintain perfect fluency. Encourage child/teen to avoid escape behaviors such as using filler words, word substitutions, and loss of eye contact, and to disclose that they stutter. The goal is to stutter more easily.
Step 4	Child/teen responds and initiates using words, phrases, sentences, and spontaneous verbal output. Voice is audible. It is important for children or teens who stutter to learn about how voice and speech are produced, and how to stutter with greater ease, including voluntary stuttering.

Note: *Parents or guardian may be part of the follow-up sessions, as determined.

When working with people who stutter, we want to take the mystery out of stuttering, and we want to consider the components that make up stuttering. The iceberg analogy is worth introducing because it takes into consideration the child/teen's dysfluent behaviors and concealment or hidden emotions. They typically focus on their repetitions, blocks, and prolongations of speech. However, avoidance and feelings of guilt and shame need to be considered. Those feelings, when disclosed, are often easier to diminish (Sheehan, 1970).

Process of Vocal Control

To vocalize, the respiratory, phonatory, and resonatory systems must work cohesively. The respiratory system (air from lungs) provides the fuel to get the voice started. The phonatory system (sound from the vocal folds or voice box) uses the airflow to set the vocal folds into vibration and to change the pitch (high and low/deep voice). The resonatory system shapes the voice into speech sounds that can come out of the mouth as in the sound /a/ as in apple, or via the nose as in the sound /m/ as in milk. Another aspect of voice production is that it can be produced reflexively/involuntarily (like when one coughs, cries, laughs, or screams) or purposefully/voluntarily (like when one produces sounds to form words for speech purposes).

When one speaks, one must be able to turn the voice ON and OFF depending on the sound the person is attempting to produce. For example, the sound /s/ as in *soap* does not use voice from the vocal folds. As one holds that sound, one only hears air coming out of the mouth. The sound /m/ as in milk requires vibrations from the vocal folds and through the nasopharynx with sound coming from the nose. Vibrations can be felt on the throat and on the nose. Timely voice initiation and good ability to turn the voice ON and OFF are necessary for adequate vocal control during speech production.

Voluntary and involuntary voice production are controlled by two different parts of the brain. For the purpose of this module, the focus will be on voluntary voice production. Voluntary voice production is essential for the initiation of speech. It is the responsibility of the anterior cingulate cortex (ACC) which translates intentions into actions, that is, it helps to provide vocal control for speech purposes (Paus, 2001). It is a specialized area of the brain that learns and adapts over time (Allman et al., 2006). The ACC plays an important role in initiation, motivation, and goal-directed behaviors. It is essential and crucial in the voluntary initiation of speech and vocalization via connections with brainstem nuclei that control the muscles of articulation and phonation (Jürgens, 2009; Medford & Critchley, 2010). According to Holroyd and Yeung (2012), the ACC shares connections with limbic structures and serves as a bridge between the decision-making process of the frontal lobe and the "emotional" world of the limbic system. Besides its role in voluntary vocal control, this part of the brain also integrates cognitive and emotional processing including anxiety (Caruana et al., 2018; Yamasaki et al., 2002). It plays an important role in regulating cognitive control over goal-directed behavior (Shenhav et al., 2013; Sheth et al., 2012). According to Shang et al. (2014), anxiety has a direct effect on the ACC as demonstrated by reductions in the right anterior cingulate gyrus and the left inferior frontal gyrus gray matter volumes, in patients with anxiety disorders. A compromised ACC lacks the ability to adequately perform its role of translating intentions into voluntary actions, and of regulating and monitoring distractors to ensure production of the intended target sound (Piai et al., 2013). Therefore, when people are uncomfortable within a situation where they are expected to speak, it becomes more difficult to purposefully initiate their voices for speech purposes (Ruiz & Klein, 2014, 2018).

Children and adolescents with selective mutism or those who stutter have difficulty initiating voice with ease for speaking. Research indicates difficulty with tension in the laryngeal area (Ruiz & Klein, 2014). Children and teens with selective mutism have identified this problem that impedes their ability to get their voice started to speak.

Using sEMG (surface electromyography), we have identified laryngeal tension during silent periods in children with selective mutism (Ruiz & Klein, 2018). Level of tension, identified by placing sensors on the individual's neck, was significantly above normal levels in children with selective mutism when asked to imitate a vowel sound or asked to say their name. By instituting a humming sound (directing voice through the nasopharynx—nose—instead of the oropharynx—mouth), we have been able to "turn the voice on" for modification of vocal control.

Success With Vocal Control

The vocal control approach has been helpful with people with selective mutism or those who stutter (PWS). We have used the vocal control approach with 42 children and adolescents who have come to the University Community Clinic for speech-language evaluations for selective mutism (Ruiz & Klein, 2018). Approximately 93% of the children were able to initiate their voices with increased ease. PWS have been reported to have longer vocal reaction times, suggesting difficulty in rapidly updating their speech/voice plans (Mock et al., 2015). The systematic and hierarchical methodology of the vocal control approach addresses reported vocal reaction time issues for people who stutter. Central control abnormalities in stuttering are a system dysfunction that interferes with rapid and dynamic speech/voice processing for production (Ludlow, 2005; Ludlow & Loucks, 2003; Ward, 2017). According to Watkins, Smith, Davis, and Howell (2008), "stuttering is a disorder related primarily to disruption in the cortical and subcortical neural systems supporting the selection, initiation and execution of motor sequences necessary for fluent speech production" (p. 50). Stuttering tends to be cyclic and difficult to irradicate completely once it becomes chronic. Vulnerabilities for chronic stuttering include social anxiety (Messenger et al., 2004) and the disruptions in the speech motor system (Kleinow & Smith, 2000). Attempts to stutter more easily and reduce escape behaviors instead of "trying to fix stuttering" are worthwhile.

Purposeful vocalizations and verbalizations may also be further compromised by our interpretations of others' emotions. According to Caballero and Díaz (2019), emotional expressions influence peoples' expectations for social decision-making, even if they have not experienced a similar interaction. Social interactions are closely dependent on our ability to decode cues and effectively respond to emotional information carried in the human voice (Grossmann et al., 2013; Hawk et al., 2009). Lima (2019) reported that individuals are able to recognize emotions within the first 500 ms of exposure of hearing someone's voice, with 90%-plus accuracy. This module dedicates a section on establishing the individual's performance for recognition, imitation, and reproduction of emotions related to voice.

To implement the skills and work toward attaining these goals, there are seven interactive activities/games, also available online for teletherapy. The companion website to access these online activities can be found in the manual.

Activity Game 1: Sound Off

This activity has three parts: (1) Nasal vs. Oral Sounds, (2) Placement and Distinctive Features of Sounds, and (3) Identification of Sound Production in Words.

Goals

- To increase awareness of nasal vs. oral and throat speech sound production.
- To increase awareness of voicing and distinctive features (nasal/oral/throat, airflow continuation or stop, voice vibration or no vibration) for speech sound production.
- To increase awareness of articulatory contacts (lips, teeth, palate, tongue, or glottal) for speech sound production.
- To identify voicing and distinctive features for speech sound production in words.

When we speak, we usually focus on the words that come out of our mouths but very little on what it takes to produce them. This section details each of the sounds in English by describing where we produce them (lips, front-mid-back of the tongue, teeth, roof of the mouth, etc.) and how we produce them (with voice, without voice, ability to hold the sound, etc.).

Anatomical illustrations are provided to aid visualization of the structures within the oral and nasal cavities. Practice sheets, found in the tables, are available to assess initial understanding of the concepts introduced in this section.

Note: Letters in brackets or slashes should be said as the sounds they make, for example, /s/ is to be said as "ssssss" and not the name of the letter "es" or /b/ is to be said as "b" and not the name of the letter "be." This is important to differentiate the concepts of airflow and voicing.

Materials: Nasal Sounds vs. Oral Sounds vs. Throat Sounds

These three categories of sounds are used to simplify speech that is produced in the nasal cavity from that produced in the back of the mouth (velars) from all other consonant sounds in English. These groupings tend to be easier for children and teens to differentiate. Illustrations showing the pathway for nasal (nose) sounds production (/m/ as in *mom*, /n/ as in *no*, and /ng/ as in *king*) (Figure 1–1).

- Illustrations showing pathway for oral (through mouth) sounds production. All vowels, all consonants except /m/, /n/, and /ng/ are primarily directed through the oral cavity (Figure 1–2).
- Illustrations showing pathway for oral/throat (back of mouth) sounds production: /k/, /g/ and /ng/, and /h/ (Figure 1–3).
- Illustrations showing all contact points of articulation for all sounds in English (Figure 1–4).

How to Play: Nasal vs. Oral and Throat Sounds

Nasal Sounds

To feel the nasal sounds, place two fingers over one side of the nose. Produce and hold the sound /m/. Feel the vibrations. Sound is traveling through the nose. Emphasis is placed on differentiating mouth from nose sounds by feeling the vibration on the nose. In order to produce these sounds, have the child/teen close their mouth and only allow the sound to come through their nose.

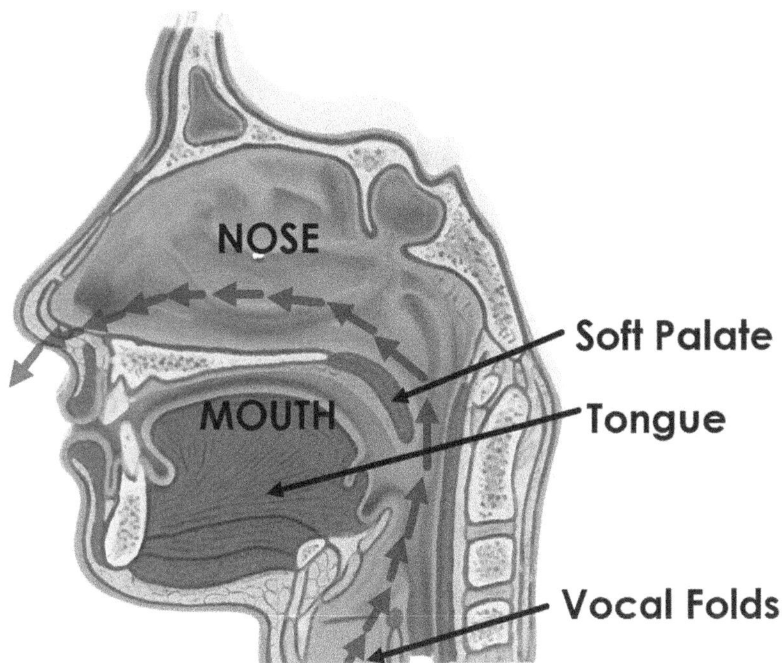

FIGURE 1–1. Nasal sounds pathway.

- Have the child/teen place their index finger on one side of their nose where the bone is and produce and hold the sound /m/ as in *mommy*. Ask the child/teen if they feel the nose vibration. Now have them try /n/ as in *nose* and "ng" as in *king*. They should still feel the nose vibrating.
- Now have them place their hands on one side of the larynx and produce the hum again. Ask the child/teen if vibration/voice is felt in the throat. Vibrations from nasal sounds are felt in both the throat (vocal cords) and the nose.

Oral Sounds

Ask the child/teen to keep their fingers on the nose and hold sounds like "ah" as in *apple* or "s" as in *soap*. They will no longer feel vibrations there because the sounds are now coming out of the mouth. The main focus is on differentiating oral and nasal sounds and becoming more aware of the trajectory of airflow and vocal vibrations. Emphasis is on the structures used for a particular sound, and whether one can feel vibration from the vocal cords (voice/no voice). Ask the child/teen to pay close attention to how much effort some sounds may require when compared to others. For example, the sound "s" as in *sip* requires less effort than the sound "ch" as in *chip*. These differences may account for variations for ease of production.

- Produce any vowel sound (not the letter) like "a" as in *apple*, "o" as in *old*, "eh" as in *elf*, and so on. They are all oral/mouth sounds.
- Produce any consonant, "p" as in *pet*, "s" as in *soap*, "k" as in *kite*, "z" as in *zoo*, "b" as in *bear*, and "g" as in *goat*. All consonants except for nasal ones like "m," "n," and "ng" come out of the mouth instead of the nose.

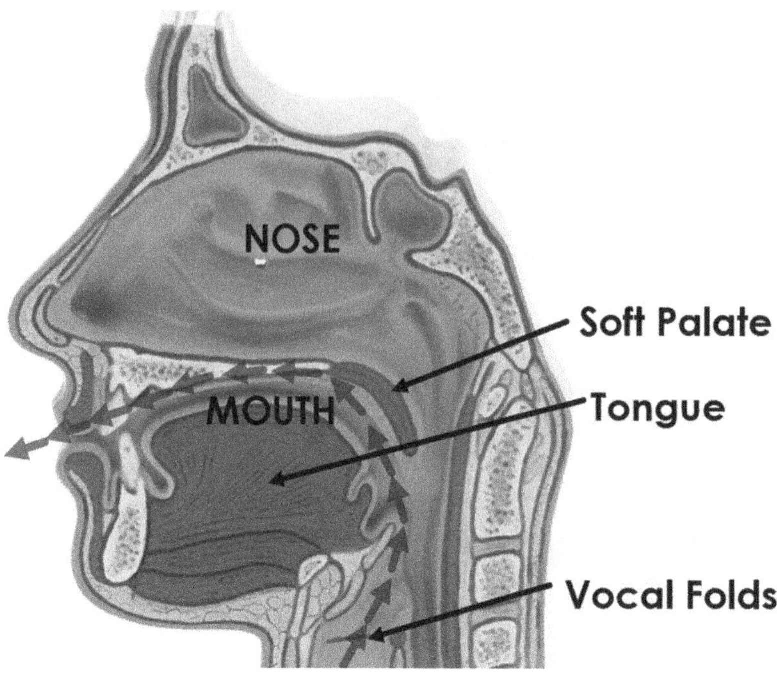

FIGURE 1–2. Oral sounds pathway.

- Some consonants are quiet because they do not use voice. They just use air. For example, the sound /s/ as in *soap* only uses air without voice, whereas the sound /z/ as in *zoo* uses the voice. To identify the difference, have the child/teen place a hand on the one side of larynx (at the Adam's apple). Hold the sound /s/, ask child/teen if vibration/voice is felt or not. Now repeat the same process with the sound /z/. When vibration is felt, voice is present, and the vocal cords are vibrating. If not, the vocal cords are not vibrating, and only air is coming out with the consonant sound.

Throat Sounds

This section focuses on sounds that are produced back in the mouth like /g/ as in *goat*, /k/ as in *cat*, and glottal /h/ as in *happy*. These sounds come out of the mouth but require increased effort to be produced; therefore, we are referring to them as *throat sounds*. If the child/teen feels uncomfortable in a situation and has difficulty initiating voice to produce a sound, those sounds that require more effort become more difficult to produce. Learning how they are produced will enhance their ability to produce the sounds when needed, despite tension. Becoming aware of the tension can help the individual learn to release it. For individuals who stutter, it can be helpful to use strategies such as light bounces for easy stuttering, and also contrast more and less tension during sound production practice. Have the child/teen practice these three sounds: /g/ as in *goat*, /k/ as in *kite*, and /h/ as in *hot*.

They are produced in the back of the mouth toward the throat.

- Have the child/teen say the word "*go*" and pay attention to where and how that sound is being produced. Now contrast it with /s/ in *soap*. The child/teen should feel the difference.

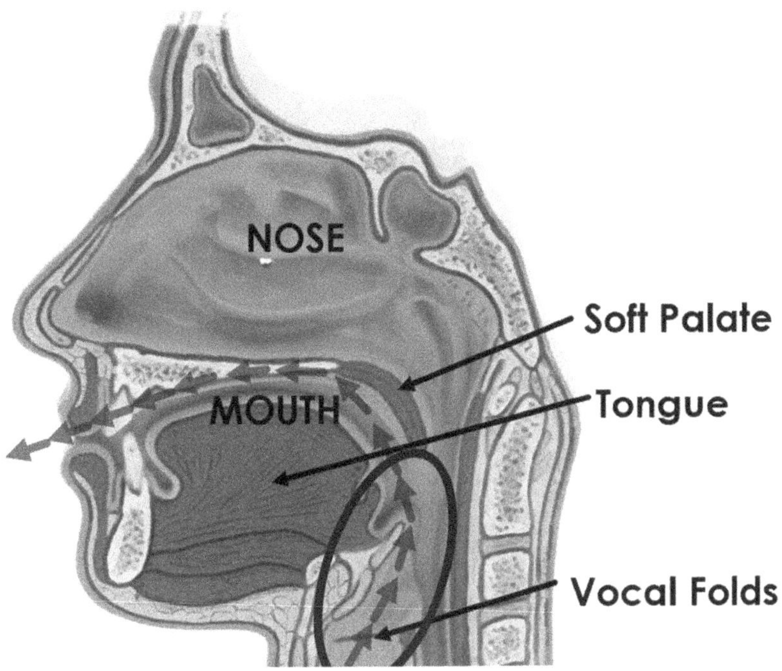

FIGURE 1–3. Oral/throat sounds pathway.

- Have the child/teen produce "g" as in the word *game* a few times and feel the back of their tongue move.
- Now have them do the same with "k" as in *cat* and "ng" as in *king*.
- Follow up by having the child/teen place their hand on their neck. Identify the sounds (not names of letters) that have vibration/voice when the child/teen produces them. Is it "k," "g," "ng," "h," or all four?
- The child/teen can move on to the next level once they correctly identify at least 8 of 10 trial sounds. The facilitator may adjust the trials accordingly.

Materials: Placement and Distinctive Features of Sounds

- Placement and Distinctive Features of Sounds (Table 1–4)

How to Play: Placement and Distinctive Features of Sounds

- Have the child/teen pay attention to the place (where the sound is produced in the mouth, in other words, what two parts are touching to make the sound) and distinctive features (how the sound is made, for example, does air keep flowing as in the sounds /s/ or /f/, or does the air stop as in /t/ or /b/). It is important that they understand that vibration for making sounds can be felt not just from the neck area but also the nose.
- Ask the child/teen to produce the underlined sounds shown in Table 1–4 (not the letter's name but the sound it makes in the word), choose where and how each sound is made and complete the chart. Table 1–5 has the answers.

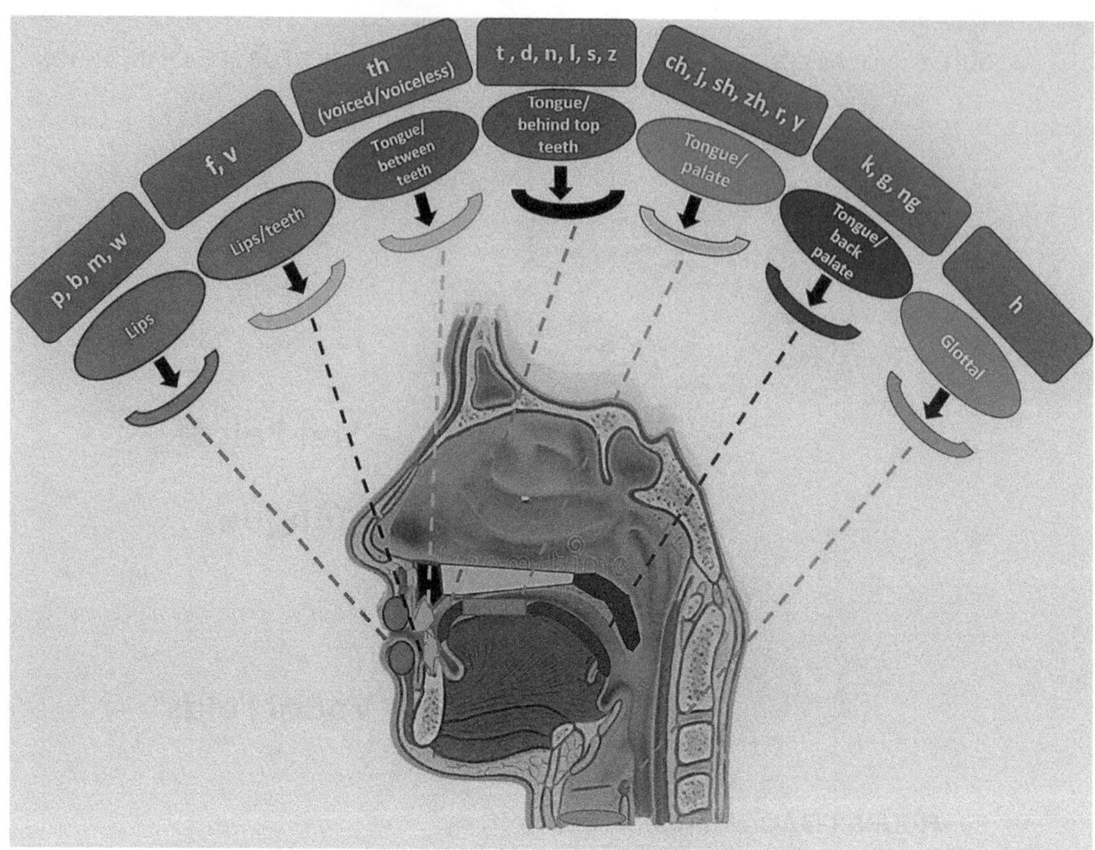

FIGURE 1–4. Contact points of articulation.

TABLE 1–4. Placement and Distinctive Features of Sounds

	Sound (nasal-oral-throat)	Airflow (continuation or stop)	Voice (vibration, no vibration)	Contact Points (lips, teeth, palate, tongue, glottal)
Leaf				
Game				
Coat				
Rose				
Wish				
Nest				
Tail				
Stop				
Dog				
King				

TABLE 1–5. Review of Speech Sound Production Chart

CONSONANTS	Mouth	Nose	Throat	Continues	Stops	Voiced	Voice-less	Contact Points
/b/ (box)	X				X	X		Lips
/d/ (dog)	X				X	X		Tongue/behind top teeth
/f/ (foot)	X			X			X	Lip/teeth
/g/ (do**g**, **g**oat)			X		X	X		Tongue/back palate
/h/ (hello)			X		X		X	Glottal
/j/ (yes)	X			X		X		Tongue/palate
/k/ (**c**oat, **k**ite)			X		X		X	Tongue/back palate
/l/ (**l**eaf, **l**ake)	X			X		X		Tongue/behind top teeth
/m/ (ga**m**e, **m**oney)		X		X		X		Lips
/n/ (**n**est, **n**o)		X		X		X		Tongue/behind top teeth
/p/ (pet)	X				X		X	Lips
/r/ (**r**ose, **r**ock)	X			X		X		Tongue/palate
/s/ (**s**top, **s**oap)	X			X			X	Tongue/behind top teeth
/t/ (**t**ail, **t**op)	X				X		X	Tongue/behind top teeth
/v/ (Vest)	X			X		X		Lip/teeth
/w/ (we)	X			X		X		Lips
/z/ (zoo)	X			X		X		Tongue/behind top teeth
/ŋ/ (ki**ng**, so**ng**)		X	X	X		X		Tongue/back palate
/ð/ (**th**at)	X			X		X		Tongue/ between teeth
/θ/ (**th**in)	X			X			X	Tongue/ between teeth
/tʃ/ (**ch**air)	X				X		X	Tongue/palate
/dʒ/ (juice)	X				X	X		Tongue/palate
/ʃ/ (wi**sh**, **sh**oe)	X			X		X		Tongue/palate

continues

TABLE 1–5. *continued*

VOWELS	Mouth				Voiced		
/ɑ/ (apple)	X				X		
/o/ (old)	X				X		
/ʊ/ (up)	X				X		
/ɛ/ (elf)	X				X		
/ɪ/ (ink)	X				X		

Materials: Identification of Sound Production in Words

- Review of Speech Sound Production Chart (Table 1–5)
- The Sound Production Board Game (Figure 1–5)
- A dice
- A timer

How to Play: Identification of Sound Production in Words

This section focuses on determining the child/teen's knowledge about sound production through activity games. The Review of Speech Sound Production Chart (Table 1–5) summarizing *where* and *how* the sounds are produced will help to reference the information at a glance, if needed. Thinking about the sounds and all that is needed to produce them will help the child/teen to focus on articulation of sounds rather than on the situation that is making them uncomfortable. Remind the child/teen that this is not a test but rather a way to practice and learn.

- Start the timer if desired.
- Have the child/teen roll the dice and move the marker to the corresponding place.
- Ask the child/teen to produce the sound at the place the marker landed, identify the placement (what areas are touching), if it is a nose or mouth or throat sound, if the airflow is continuous or stop, and whether it is voiced or voiceless. If working on modifying tension, use the timer as this makes the task more challenging.
- Child/teen collects the number of points listed under each word.
- Child/teen should continue rolling the dice until making it all the way around to the start line.
- Stop the timer once child/teen makes it back to the starting line.
- Record the amount of time it took and add the number of points collected.
- Depending on how difficult the task is for the child/teen, they should be encouraged to challenge themselves with another round and try beating their own time record.
- Points collected may be deposited in a bank to be used toward obtaining an agreed upon item/award.

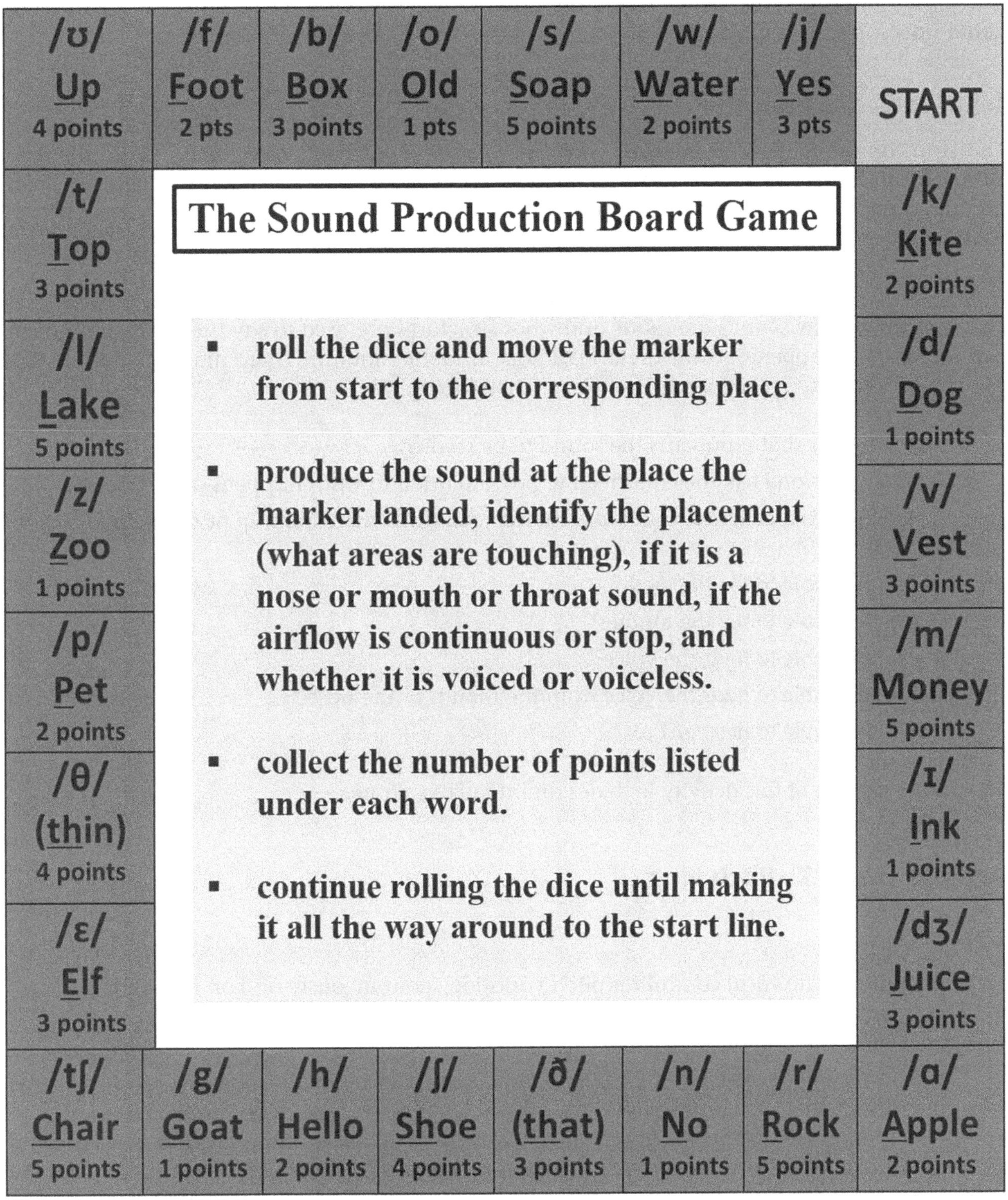

/ʊ/ Up 4 points	/f/ Foot 2 pts	/b/ Box 3 points	/o/ Old 1 pts	/s/ Soap 5 points	/w/ Water 2 points	/j/ Yes 3 pts	START
/t/ Top 3 points							/k/ Kite 2 points
/l/ Lake 5 points							/d/ Dog 1 points
/z/ Zoo 1 points							/v/ Vest 3 points
/p/ Pet 2 points							/m/ Money 5 points
/θ/ (thin) 4 points							/ɪ/ Ink 1 points
/ɛ/ Elf 3 points							/dʒ/ Juice 3 points
/tʃ/ Chair 5 points	/g/ Goat 1 points	/h/ Hello 2 points	/ʃ/ Shoe 4 points	/ð/ (that) 3 points	/n/ No 1 points	/r/ Rock 5 points	/ɑ/ Apple 2 points

The Sound Production Board Game

- **roll the dice and move the marker from start to the corresponding place.**
- **produce the sound at the place the marker landed, identify the placement (what areas are touching), if it is a nose or mouth or throat sound, if the airflow is continuous or stop, and whether it is voiced or voiceless.**
- **collect the number of points listed under each word.**
- **continue rolling the dice until making it all the way around to the start line.**

FIGURE 1–5. The sound production board game.

Apps to Consider

If able, the facilitator can get the apps discussed in the following sections to help learn more about how sounds are produced

Small Talk—Phonemes

This app can be obtained from *https://www.aphasia.com/smalltalk-aphasia-apps/*. Go to the App Store on the iPhone or iPad. Type in *Small talk phonemes* to get it. This app shows a person producing each consonant and vowel sound in English.

Speech Tutor From speechtutor.org

This app shows how sounds are made and what structures are used to say them. The child/teen can see what is happening with the articulators inside the mouth. There may be a fee for this app. Open either app. For Speech Tutor select the *video* option.

- Select a letter that represents the sound to be studied.
- See the video and ask the child/teen to pay attention to what happens at the mouth:
  - Are the lips together or apart, are they spread (like when smiling) or rounded (as when puckering)?
  - Are they able to see the teeth?
  - Are they able to see the tongue?
  - Are they able to hear the voice?
  - Are they able to hear the voice from the mouth or the nose?
  - Are they able to hear just air?

The online version of this activity includes an interactive game.

Activity Game 2: Pitch Pipe

Goals

- To demonstrate vocal control for pitch variation spontaneously and on demand
- To discuss the concept of high and low voice by demonstrating the differences

The child/teen has learned how sounds are produced and whether they have voice (vocal cords vibrating) or not. Now it is time to learn how the pitch of the voice can be changed from high to low or low to high. Being able to change the pitch helps to let others know whether one is asking a question (raising pitch at the end of the sentence) or ending a statement (lowering pitch at the end of the sentence). Sometimes when one feels too much neck tension, it is difficult to change the pitch. Being able to change the pitch purposefully can be helpful to relax the voice when it becomes too tight to be produced.

Materials

- Timer
- Pitch pipe or Pocket Pitch (https://apps.apple.com/us/app/pocket-pitch-the-singer-app/id1005725401)
- One deck of cards labeled with *high*, *normal*, and *low* (four each) (Table 1–6)
- One deck of cards labeled with pictures (person, place, or object) (12 total) (Figure 1–6)

Copy Figure 1–6 and cut off each picture to form 12 different cards. Use the cards to play the game as instructed on the activity game 2 (Pitch Pipe)—Level 2.

How to Play

Level 1

- Play a tone using the pitch pipe or the app Pocket Pitch (https://apps.apple.com/us/app/pocket-pitch-the-singer-app/id1005725401) or similar.
- Have the child/teen imitate the pitch provided. The idea is to have the child/teen learn to vary pitch rather than to have a perfect match.
- Once the child/teen has successfully approximated 8 out of 10 pitch trials presented, they can move to the next level. The number of trials can be adjusted accordingly.

Level 2

- Make two stacks of cards. One with pitch words on Table 1–6, and the other with pictures on Figure 1–6.
- Have the child/teen pick a card from the pitch word stack to use when they say the name of the picture (in the other stack of cards).
- Ask the child/teen to name the picture at the pitch level described.
- Once the child/teen is comfortable with the activity, the facilitator can try doing this activity against the clock. The more words said at the designated pitch in 15 seconds, the better. Time can be adjusted accordingly.

Apps to Consider

- Pocket Pitch (https://apps.apple.com/us/app/pocket-pitch-the-singer-app/id1005725401) to hear different pitches.
- SpinnyWheel (Brain Clippings) (https://apps.apple.com/us/app/spinnywheel/id901444671) to help the facilitator randomize the different pitches the child/teen needs to produce. Once downloaded, add the words *high*, *low*, and *normal* to the choices, following the instruction in the app. Have the child/teen spin the wheel so they know what pitch to use when they name the picture.

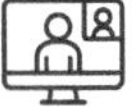
The online version of this activity includes an interactive game.

Activity Game 3: Ramp It Up!

Goals

- To demonstrate vocal control for loudness variation spontaneously and on demand
- To discuss the concept of loud and soft voice by demonstrating the differences

Another aspect of voice is how loud or how soft it can be produced. Sometimes one may need to yell; other times one may need to speak very softly as if telling a secret. Learning to change the loudness is helpful to continue to gain control of the voice. Increasing loudness requires that more air flows through the vocal folds. When the throat tightens up, it is more difficult to make the voice louder. The ability to change loudness also promotes vocal cord and throat relaxation and control. When an individual pairs these skills with the ability to change pitch, the voice is produced more easily.

Materials

- Timer
- Deck of cards labeled *soft, normal, loud,* and *whisper* (Table 1–7)
- Deck of cards with pictures on each card (Figure 1–6)
- Decibel X (SkyPaw Co.) (https://apps.apple.com/us/app/decibel-x-db-sound-level-meter/id448155923) or similar apps
- Speak Up Too (Sensory App House) (https://apps.apple.com/us/app/speak-up-too-speech-fun/id922513159)
- Bla Bla Bla (Lorenzo Bravi) (https://apps.apple.com/us/app/bla-bla-bla/id430815432)

How to Play

Level 1

- Have the child/teen count while *increasing* loudness. For example, ONE in a *soft* voice, TWO in a *normal* loudness, and THREE in a *medium-loud* loudness, and FOUR in a *very loud* loudness.
- Count while *decreasing* loudness. For example, ONE in a *very loud* voice, TWO in a *medium* loudness, THREE in a *normal* loudness, and FOUR in a *soft* voice.

Level 2

- Pick a card from the stack of cards labeled *soft, normal, loud,* and *whisper.*
- Have the child/teen pick a card from the loudness word stack to use when they say the name of the picture (in the other stack of cards).
- Ask the child/teen to name the picture (Figure 1–6) at the loudness level described (Table 1–7).
- Once the child/teen is comfortable with the activity, the facilitator can try doing this activity against the clock. The more words said at the designated pitch in 15 seconds, the better. Time can be adjusted accordingly.

TABLE 1–6. Pitch Words

Copy this page and cut off each word to form 12 different cards. Mix them up and use the cards to play the game as instructed on the Activity Game 2 (Pitch Pipe)—Level 2.

HIGH	NORMAL	LOW
HIGH	NORMAL	LOW
HIGH	NORMAL	LOW
HIGH	NORMAL	LOW

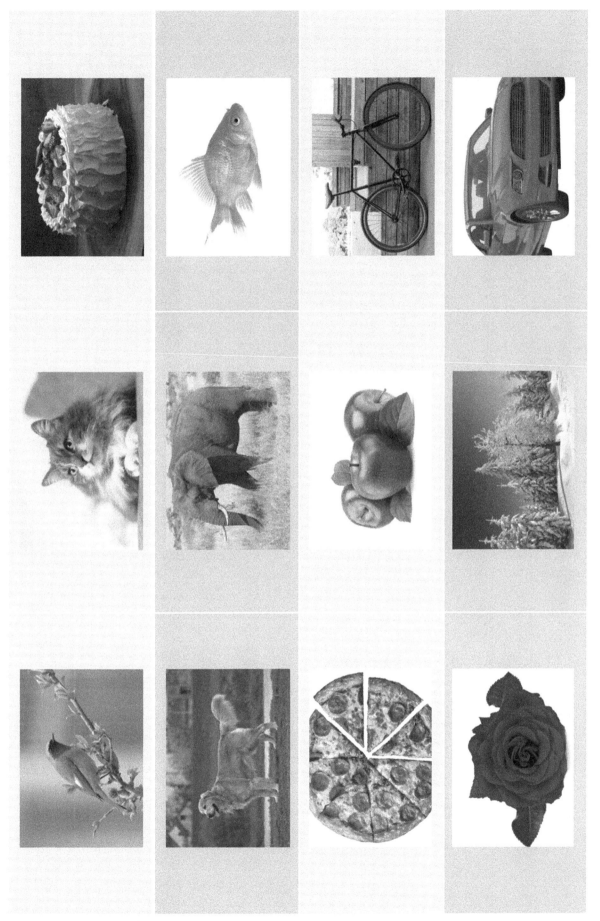

FIGURE 1–6. Pictures for activity games 2 and 3.

TABLE 1–7. Loudness Words

Copy this page and cut off each word to form 12 different cards. Mix them up and use the cards to play the game as instructed on Activity Game 3: Ramp It Up!			
SOFT	NORMAL	LOUD	WHISPER
SOFT	NORMAL	LOUD	WHISPER
SOFT	NORMAL	LOUD	WHISPER

Apps to Consider

The loudness can be monitored by using the following apps:

- Decibel X (SkyPaw Co.) (https://apps.apple.com/us/app/decibel-x-db-sound-level-meter/id448155923) is a sound loudness meter. Normal voice with the phone at 3 feet from the child/teen should be about 65 dB, less than 55 dB is soft, 70 to 80 dB is loud, and greater than 80 dB is very loud.
- Speak Up Too (Sensory App House) (https://apps.apple.com/us/app/speak-up-too-speech-fun/id922513159) provides color visual images that change depending on loudness level.
- Bla Bla Bla (Lorenzo Bravi) (https://apps.apple.com/us/app/bla-bla-bla/id430815432) provides black-and-white visual images of faces that change depending on loudness level.

For randomization of the loudness words, the following app can be used:

- Use the app SpinnyWheel (Brain Clippings) (https://apps.apple.com/us/app/spinnywheel/id901444671) with the words *soft*, *normal*, *loud*, and *whisper* following the instruction in the app. Have the child/teen spin the wheel and be ready to name the picture at the loudness shown by the wheel once it stops.

The online version of this activity includes an interactive game.

Activity Game 4: Vocal Marathon

Goals

- To discuss the concept of freeing the voice via easy voice onset from humming /m/ and /h/ initiated words to speech
- To increase vocal ability to sustain the voice for 5 to 10 seconds, as able

So far, the child/teen has learned that when speaking, sounds are produced in different places including the nose and the mouth. They also learned that some sounds have voice while others do not, some can be prolonged and others not, and that pitch and loudness can be changed as needed. Now the child/teen is ready to use those skills to start moving from vocalizations to verbalizations, that is, from sounds to initiation of speech. Humming is the most relaxed sound one can produce. It maintains all structures at their relaxed state and comes from the nose.

Another sound that promotes reduction of tension in the neck or larynx is the sound /h/ as in *happy*. This sounds prevents the vocal cords from closing and keeps air flowing. This section focuses on using those two sounds (/m/ and /h/) with syllables and words.

Materials

- Timer.
- Bla Bla Bla (Lorenzo Bravi) (https://apps.apple.com/us/app/bla-bla-bla/id430815432) provides black-and-white visual images of faces that change depending on loudness level.
- Random /m/ words (Table 1–8).
- Random /h/ words (Table 1–9).
- Random /m/ sentences (Table 1–10).
- Random /h/ sentences (Table 1–11).

How to Play

Level 1: Humming

- Have the child/teen prolong a hum for at least 5 to 10 seconds while feeling how relaxing it is to produce a hum. Increments may be needed until reaching the goal of 10 seconds.
- Ask the child/teen to put a finger on the side of their nose on the bone to make sure the hum is coming out the nose.
- Once the child/teen can make a relaxed hum, they can move to the next task. To do this, initiate the Bla Bla Bla app (https://apps.apple.com/us/app/bla-bla-bla/id430815432).
- Choose the face of one of the characters. Have the child/teen put their finger on their neck (Adam's apple) to feel the vibration of the vocal cords as they make the humming sound. Make the humming /m/ into the Bla Bla Bla app, as quietly as possible. The app picks up sound; the louder the sound, the more expression there is on the faces of characters. Try to have the child/teen produce the /m/ sound quietly enough so that the vocal cords vibrate but the characters' faces on the app do not activate. The purpose is for easy onset of voice production that can be built upon.

Level 2: Humming to Vowels

- Have the child/teen initiate a comfortable hum and change it into a vowel like /a/ as in *mom* without stopping the voice. (e.g., mmmmmmmmmaaaaaaaaaaaaaaaah).
- Ask the child/teen to prolong the vowel for 5 to 10 seconds while maintaining an easy and relaxed voice.
- Repeat the /m/ into other vowels as described (ah, oh, eeh, oo, eh). Remember the goal is at least 5 to 10 seconds, but the longer the better. Increments may be needed until reaching the goal of 10 seconds.

Additional Apps to Consider

Have the child/teen use humming and/or vowels to activate and play the games.

- Scream Note Games (Sang Mobile) (https://play.google.com/store/apps/details?id=com.sanggames.eighthnote&hl=en_US&gl=US) It is good for gaining control of the voice to move and jump between platforms.

TABLE 1–8. Random /m/ Words

Copy this page and cut off each word to form 24 different cards. Use the cards to play the game as instructed on the Activity Game 4—Level 3.

MONEY	MILK	MELON
MOVIE	MUSIC	MEAT
MALL	MANAGER	MAN
MOON	MARCH	MAGIC
MARKET	MAY	MEAL
MOTHER	MENU	METAL
MEDICAL	MEMORY	MIDDLE
MIRROR	MINUTE	MISTAKE

TABLE 1–9. Random /h/ Words

Copy this page and cut off each word to form 24 different cards. Use the cards to play the game as instructed on the Activity Game 4—Level 3.		
HAIR	HAMMER	HALF
HAND	HAPPY	HARD
HAT	HANDLE	HEAD
HEAL	HEALTH	HEAR
HEAVY	HELLO	HEEL
HELP	HEART	HERO
HIGH	HINT	HISTORY
HOBBY	HIGHWAY	HEADACHE

TABLE 1–10. Random /m/ Sentences

Copy this table and use it to play the game as instructed on Activity Game 4—Level 6.
My mother makes marvelous meatballs.
Michelle missed my message.
Mary Morgan makes me mad.
Mike's mechanical men make microphones.
My mother makes me miss many movies.
Molly Mitchell makes mystery movies.
Movies make me miss my mom.
Marci made many magic machines.
My mother makes me mind my manners.
Michael married my mother's maid.

TABLE 1–11. Random /h/ Sentences

Copy this table and use it to play the game as instructed on Activity Game 4—Level 6.
Harry helps him.
His horse has hooves.
He hates hot honey.
Harold has handkerchiefs.
He hopes he has help.
Hannah has honey hotcakes.
Hoppity hop hop hop.
Harvey has heavy hands.
Holly's hat helps hide her hair.
He hit his head hard.

Level 3: From /m/ and /h/ to Words

- Have the child/teen start by warming up the voice by holding a hum for a minimum of 5 to 10 seconds at three different times.
- Cut the 24 /m/ words from Table 1–8. Place a stack of the 24 /m/ words (which is the same sound as a hum) face down in front of the child/teen (e.g., milk, music, etc.). Set the timer to 10 seconds. Start the timer and have the child/teen begin to pick one card at the time and say the /m/ word as soon as they see it. This adds an element of expectation and fun that can benefit the child/teen with selective mutism as they learn to control their voice. See how many they can read/say before the time is up. For the child/teen who stutters, this strategy supports easy onset of phonation in a game-like manner.
- Repeat the activity again but this time using the /h/ initiated words (see Table 1–9).

Level 4: Generating /m/ Words

- Now give the child/teen 1 minute to *name as many words as possible* that start with /m/.
- Start the timer and have the child/teen begin saying the words.
- Count how many words after 1 minute. Adding a time constraint in a practice format can help desensitize time pressure during speech.
- When appropriate, challenge the child/teen to break their own record.
- When comfortable with this task, the child/teen should repeat the activity generating /h/ words. They may prolong the /h/ sound to ease into the words as needed. If the child/teen experiences difficulty initiating the sound, they can imitate the facilitator in unison, or they can also use prolongations, repetitions, and blocks to contrast and reflect on differences in production.

Level 5: From /m/ Words to /m/ Sentences

- Ask the child/teen to read sentences that contain /m/ words (see Table 1–10).
- Allow the child/teen 15 seconds to read as many sentences as possible.
- Have the child/teen read each sentence clearly at a natural pace.
- The first time, ask the child/teen to read the sentences from top to bottom, the second time from bottom to top.
- To increase tolerance for anxiety related to speech, add a timer. Once the child/teen can read at least six sentences in the amount of time given, they are ready to move to the next activity. Depending on the child/teen, the number of sentences may need to be adjusted.

Level 6: From /h/ Words to /h/ Sentences

- Ask the child/teen to read sentences that contain /h/ words (see Table 1–11).
- Allow the child/teen 15 seconds to read as many sentences as possible.
- Have the child/teen read each sentence clearly at a natural pace.

- The first time, ask the child/teen to read the sentences from top to bottom, the second time from bottom to top.
- To increase tolerance for anxiety related to speech, add a timer. Once the child/teen can read at least six sentences in the amount of time given, they are ready to move to the next activity. Depending on the child/teen, the number of sentences may need to be adjusted.

 The online version of this activity includes an interactive game.

Activity Game 5: Tag Along Words

Goals

- To demonstrate carryover of skills by generating words from random sounds

This section focuses on using the child/teen's knowledge about sound production to generate other words. Interactive activities provide the stimuli and add a level of expectation with the option of using a timer. The more words the child/teen can produce within the time provided, the better. For those who stutter, the focus is on stuttering more easily; for those with selective mutism, the focus is on initiating vocalization. The focus is to think of a new word that begins with the final sound (not the letter) from the previous word. Using sound-symbol correspondence in this activity, both groups gain practice with generating new words using their learned skills.

Materials

- A stack of 24 cards containing random words to cut and use in Table 1–12
- A timer

How to Play

- Set and start the timer (optional).
- Ask the child/teen to pick a card from the pile.
- Ask the child/teen to say the word and to produce another word that begins with the last sound (not the letter) of the word read. For example, if the child/teen picks a card with the word BACKPACK, then they can produce the word CAT, as it begins with the sound /k/, which is the same one that BACKPACK ends with.
- Once completed, have the child/teen pick another card.
- Ask the child/teen to move through the pile. If using the timer, you can modify speed to go as quickly as possible to beat the clock or to compare times if there is another player. Be prepared to adjust the speed accordingly to accommodate the individual child/teen, if needed. For some children or teens this can be a motivator, for others it can be discouraging.
- Work toward completing all the words in the list and adding new ones as desired.

TABLE 1–12. Random Words

Copy this page and cut off each word to form 24 different cards. Use the cards to play the game as instructed on the Activity Game 5—Tag Along.

SPORTS	PHONE	CAR
GAMES	PAPER	VIDEO
SCREEN	COMPUTER	PLATE
PICTURE	SELFIE	TRIP
SMILE	TEACHER	FATHER
MOTHER	DOCTOR	SCHOOL
PRINTER	LAPTOP	iPAD
iPHONE	SHOES	WINTER

- For children/teens with selective mutism, reduce direct eye contact on the child/teen, rather focus on the word and activity.
- For children who stutter, identify how speech works and contrast fluent speech with productions of sounds where tension is felt to gain a clearer understanding of easy stuttering.

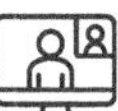 The online version of this activity includes an interactive game.

Activity Game 6: What's Up?

Goals

- To use learned strategies to initiate speech to respond to questions

Now it is time for the child/teen to use their learned skills to formulate speech to answer random questions. Answering direct questions may create anxiety or stress, especially for those who tend to be more perfectionistic and fear making a mistake. Remind them that this is not a knowledge test but rather a way to practice responding. There is no right or wrong answer. Let the child/teen know that it is OK to express when they are feeling nervous or anxious about a task. The facilitator can use this as a teachable moment to convey their own experiences and how they handle that (e.g., take a few breaths, say positive things to oneself, tense and slowly release a fist or toes). Encourage the child/teen to challenge themselves to respond using the strategies to free the voice.

Materials

- Timer (optional)
- General Questions—Single-word responses (Table 1–13)

How to Play

Level 1: Vocal Warm-Up

- Child/teen to start by warming up their voice by going through the following steps:
  - i. Hold a hum for at least 10 seconds.
  - ii. Produce 10 /h/ words, prolonging the /h/ before saying the word if needed.
  - iii. Produce 10 /m/ words while humming or prolonging the /m/ before saying the word, if needed.

Level 2: Responding to Open-Ended Questions

- Use the 21 cards with questions (Table 1–13). Copy and cut them into individual cards. Now place a stack of cards with the questions to answer in front of the child/teen.
- Have the child/teen pick a card and verbally respond to the questions.

- If there are any issues initiating the voice, remind the child/teen to use /m/ or /h/ to initiate the voice and ease into the word.
- Pick a card and ask the question to the child/teen.
- Child/teen to verbally respond to the question accordingly.
- Again, if there are any issues initiating the voice, remind the child/teen to use /m/ or /h/ to initiate and free the voice.
- Continue to take turns.
- If appropriate, challenge the child/teen to respond to a minimum of questions in a specific amount of time (e.g., 1 minute).

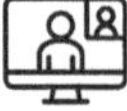 The online version of this activity includes an interactive game.

TABLE 1–13. Open-Ended Questions

Copy this page and cut off each question to form 21 different cards. Use the cards as instructed to answer the questions in Activity Game 6—What's Up?

HOW OLD DO YOU HAVE TO BE TO START DRIVING?	WHAT ARE THE COLORS OF THE U.S. FLAG?	WHY COULDN'T A BLIND PERSON DRIVE?
WHAT IS YOUR FAVORITE MOVIE?	WHAT IS YOUR BEST FRIEND'S NAME?	WHAT KIND OF THINGS DO YOU DO WITH YOUR FRIENDS?
WHO IS YOUR FAVORITE TEACHER THIS YEAR?	WHAT IS YOUR LEAST FAVORITE CLASS THIS YEAR?	WHAT IS YOUR FAVORITE LUNCH TO HAVE IN SCHOOL?
WHAT IS YOUR FAVORITE APP?	WHAT IS YOUR FAVORITE TV SHOW?	WHO IS YOUR FAVORITE CELEBRITY?
WHAT IS YOUR FAVORITE PET?	WHAT IS YOUR FAVORITE BAND?	WHAT IS YOUR FAVORITE VIDEO GAME?
WHAT IS YOUR FAVORITE SONG?	WOULD YOU RATHER BE THE BOSS OR THE EMPLOYEE?	IF YOU COULD GIVE SOMEONE A GIFT, WHO IS IT AND WHAT WOULD IT BE?
IF YOU COULD LIVE ANYWHERE IN THE WORLD, WHERE WOULD IT BE?	IF YOU COULD EAT ANY FOOD AT A RESTAURANT, WHAT WOULD YOU ORDER?	WHAT DO YOU THINK IS THE BEST JOB IN THE WORLD?

Activity Game 7: Let's Face It

Goals

- To label the emotions
- To identify emotions from vocal intonation
- To imitate the expressions and intonation to show the emotion with the voice
- To make up a sentence and use the voice to express the emotion

Our ability to initiate speech is also influenced by our interpretations of others' emotions either from their faces or their voices. This section provides practical and interactive activities to learn about the child/teen's ability to accurately label, identify, imitate, and produce emotions.

Materials

- Pictures that depict different emotions (Figures 1–7, 1–8, 1–9, 1–10, and 1–11).
- A list of sentences depicting emotions (e.g., "This is terrible. I'm so sad.") to be read to the child/teen to imitate the emotion and/or to be used by the child/teen when expressing emotions (Figure 1–12).

How to Play

Level 1: Labeling Emotions

- Use pictures (Figures 1–7, 1–8, 1–9, 1–10, and 1–11) that depict the different emotions shown on Figure 1–13.
- Have the child/teen label each of the emotions depicted.
- If child/teen is unsure, provide them with two choices to select one (e.g., angry or disgusted).

Level 2: Identifying Emotions

- Facilitator reads the sentences to the child/teen using the list of phrases or sentences that correspond to the expression of an emotion (Figure 1–12) without showing the pictures.
- Have the child/teen identify the emotion that they hear by saying the label or pointing to the corresponding picture (Figure 1–13).

Level 3: Imitating the Expressions and Intonation to Show the Emotion

- Use the sentences/phrases created for Level 2 (Figure 1–12); the online version contains recorded sentences.
- Have the child/teen imitate how you, the facilitator, sound when saying the sentences or phrases. Make sure the child/teen uses similar intonation as that which you demonstrated.

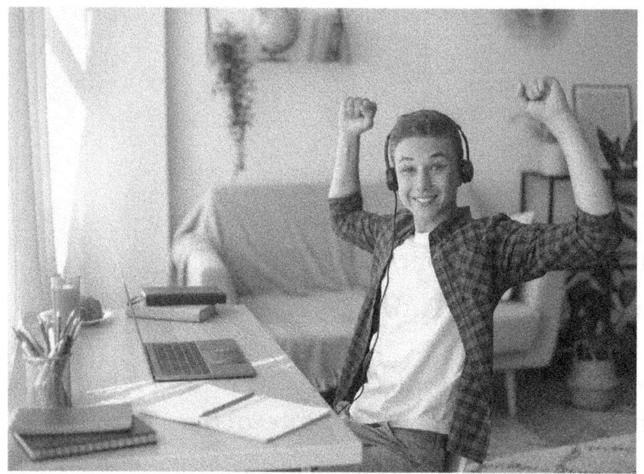

FIGURE 1–7. Happy.

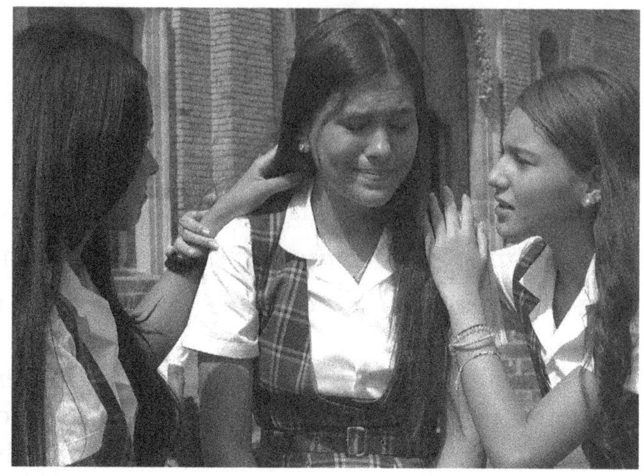

FIGURE 1–8. Sad.

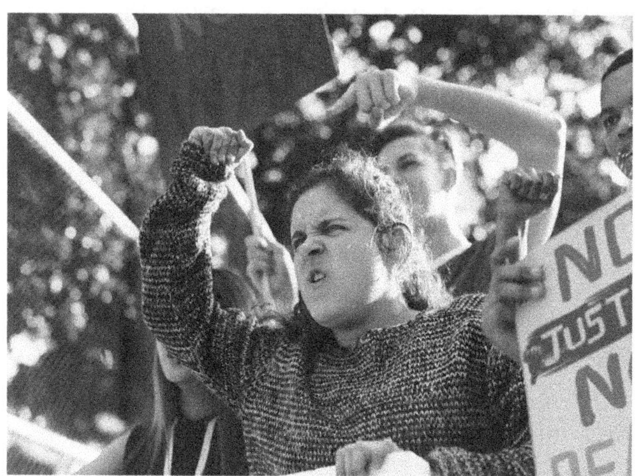

FIGURE 1–9. Angry.

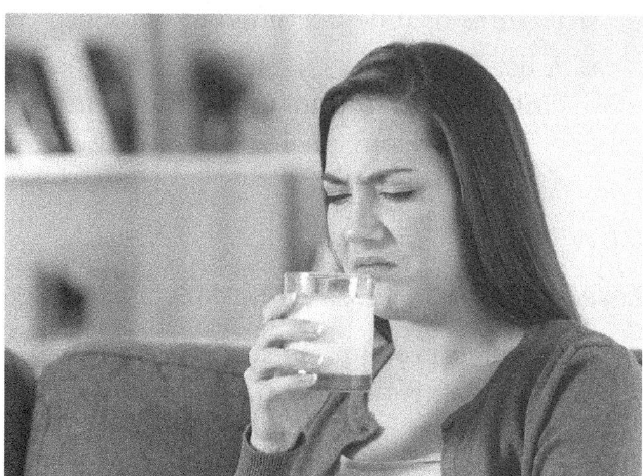

FIGURE 1–10. Disgusted.

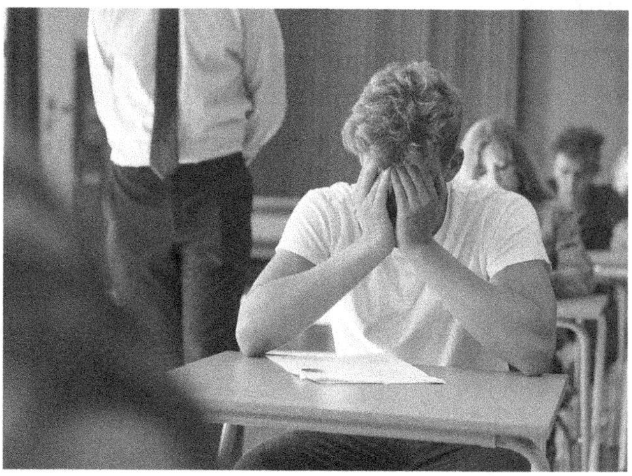

FIGURE 1–11. Anxious.

I got it. This is great! I'm so happy.

This is terrible. I'm so sad.

This is stressful. I'm worried and anxious.

I don't like this at all. It's so disgusting.

This gets me so angry.

FIGURE 1–12. Sentences to show emotions.

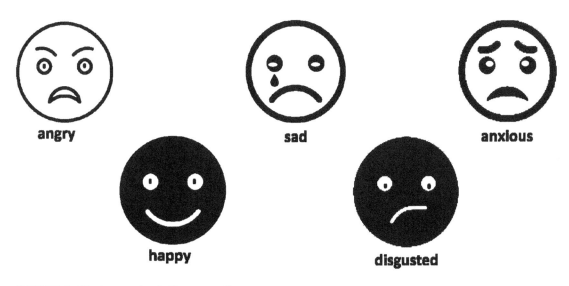

FIGURE 1–13. Icons depicting emotions.

Level 4: Producing Emotions Spontaneously

- Have the child/teen produce an emotion by saying whatever they want, to express that emotion. The child/teen may start with the phrases or sentences already said before (Figure 1–12) and continue with new sentences such as those below. Feel free to have the child/teen make up their own sentences too.
  - ☐ *Look! I just got a new phone.*
  - ☐ *Stop it, I don't like that.*
  - ☐ *I can't do the presentation tomorrow.*
  - ☐ *I'm not planning to go.*
  - ☐ *I don't like that lady, she sounded mean.*
  - ☐ *The new kid in class is cool.*
  - ☐ *I wish things were different.*
  - ☐ *How much does that cost?*
  - ☐ *I want to get one, but it's too expensive.*
  - ☐ *I just love summertime.*
  - ☐ *Do you want to meet up sometime?*
  - ☐ *Our new teacher is really nice.*
  - ☐ *I don't want to eat that!*
  - ☐ *I'm not going to the party. Are you?*
  - ☐ *Don't show me that. I don't want to see it.*
- Using the icons that depict emotions (Figure 1–13), the facilitator is to guess the emotion the child/teen is trying to convey. Make sure to emphasize to the child/teen that it is not only the words used but the intonation that goes with them.

 The online version of this activity includes an interactive game.

CONGRATULATIONS. THE CHILD/TEEN IS NOW MUCH BETTER AT FREEING AND CONTROLLING THEIR VOICE, AND READY TO MOVE TO MODULE 2.

References

Allman, J. M., Hakeem, A., Erwin, J. M., Nimchinsky, E., & Hof, P. (2006). The anterior cingulate cortex: Evolution of an interface between emotion and cognition. *Annals of the New York Academy of Sciences, 935*(1), 107–117. https://doi.org/10.1111/j.1749-6632.2001.tb03476.x

Bouchard, K. E., Mesgarani, N., Johnson, K., & Chang, E. F. (2013). Functional organization of human sensorimotor cortex for speech articulation. *Nature, 495*(21), 327–332. https://doi.org/10.1038/nature11911

Caballero, J.A., & Diaz, M.M. (2019). On the role of vocal emotions in social decision-making. *Current Psychology*. https://doi.org/10.1007/s12144-019-00509-1

Caruana, F., Gerbella, M., Avanzini, P., Gozzo, F., Pelliccia, V., Roberto, R., . . . Rizzolatti, G. (2018). Motor and emotional behaviours elicited by electrical stimulation of the human cingulate cortex, *Brain, 141*(10), 3035–3051. https://doi.org/10.1093/brain/awy219

Davis, P. J., Zhang, S. P., Winkworth, A., & Bandler, R. (1996). Neural control of vocalization: Respiratory and emotional influences. *Journal of Voice, 10*(1), 23–38.

Grossmann, T., Vaish, A., Franz, J., Schroeder, R., Stoneking, M., & Friederici, A. D. (2013). Emotional voice processing: Investigating the role of genetic variation in the serotonin transporter across development. *PLOS ONE, 8*(7), e68377. https://doi.org/10.1371/journal.pone.0068377

Hawk, S. T., van Kleef, G. A., Fischer, A. H., & van der Schalk, J. (2009). "Worth a thousand words": Absolute and relative decoding of nonlinguistic affect vocalizations. *Emotion, 9*(3), 293–305. https://doi.org/10.1037/a0015178

Holroyd, C. B., & Yeung, N. (2012). Motivation of extended behaviors by anterior cingulate cortex. *Trends in Cognitive Sciences, 16*(2), 122–128.

Jürgens, U. (2002). Neural pathways underlying vocal control. *Neuroscience & Biobehavioral Reviews, 26*(2), 235–258. https://doi.org/10.1016/S0149-7634(01)00068-9

Jürgens, U. (2009). The neural control of vocalizations in mammals: A review. *Journal of Voice, 23*(1), 2–10.

Kleinow, J., & Smith, A. (2000). Influences of length and syntactic complexity on the speech motor stability of the fluent speech of adults who stutter. *Journal of Speech, Language, and Hearing Research, 43*, 548–559.

Lima, C. F. (2019). Automaticity in the recognition of nonverbal emotional vocalizations. *Emotion, 19*(2), 219–233. http://doi.org/10.1037/emo0000429

Ludlow, C. L. (2005). Central nervous system control of the laryngeal muscles in humans. *Respiratory Physiology & Neurobiology, 147*(2–3), 205–222. https://doi.org/10.1016/j.resp.2005.04.015

Ludlow, C. L., & Loucks, T. (2003). Stuttering: A dynamic motor control disorder. *Journal of Fluency Disorders, 28*, 273–295.

Medford, N., & Critchley, H. D. (2010). Conjoint activity of anterior insular and anterior cingulate cortex: Awareness and response. *Brain Structural Function, 214*, 535–549. https://doi.org/10.1007/s00429-010-0265-x

Messenger, M., Onslow, M., Packman, A., & Menzies, R. (2004). Social anxiety in stuttering: Measuring negative social expectancies. *Journal of Fluency Disorders, 29*, 201–212.

Mock, J. R., Foundas, A. L., & Golob, E. J. (2016). Cortical activity during cued picture naming predicts individual differences in stuttering frequency. *Clinical Neurophysiology, 127*(9), 3093–3101.

Paus, T. (2001). Primate anterior cingulate cortex: Where motor control, drive and cognition interface. *Nature Reviews/Neuroscience, 2*, 417–424.

Piai, V., Roelofs, A., Acheson, D. J., & Takashima, A. (2013). Attention for speaking: Domain-general control from the anterior cingulate cortex in spoken word production. *Frontiers in Human Neuroscience, 7*(832), 1–13.

Ruiz, C., & Klein, E. R. (2014). The effects of anxiety on voice production: A retrospective case report of selective mutism. *Pennsylvania Speech-Language-Hearing Association Journal, 4*, 19–26.

Ruiz, C. E., & Klein, E. R. (2018). Surface electromyography to identify laryngeal tension in selective mutism: Could this be the missing link? *Biomedical Journal of Scientific & Technical Research, 12*(2), 1–4.

Shang, J., Fu, Y., Ren, Z., Zhang, T., Du, M,, et al. (2014). The common traits of the ACC and PFC in anxiety disorders in the DSM-5: Meta-analysis of voxelbased morphometry studies. *PLoS ONE 9*(3), e93432. https://doi.org/10.1371/journal.pone.0093432

Sheehan, J. G. (1970). *Stuttering: Research and treatment.* Harper & Row.

Shenhav, A., Botvinick, M. M., & Cohen, J. D. (2013). The expected value of control: An integrative theory of anterior cingulate cortex function. *Neuron Review, 79*, 217–240.

Sheth, S. A., Mian, M. K., Patel, S. R., Asaad, W. F., Williams, Z. M., Dougherty, D. D., . . . Eskandar, E. N. (2012). Human dorsal anterior cingulate cortex neurons mediate ongoing behavioral adaptation. *Nature, 488*(7410), 218–221.

Sisskin, V. (2018). Avoidance reduction therapy for stuttering (ARTS). In B. J. Amster & E. R. Klein (Eds.), *More than fluency: The social, emotional, and cognitive dimensions of stuttering.* Plural Publishing.

Smith, A., & Weber, C. (2017). How stuttering develops: The multifactorial dynamic pathways theory. *Journal of Speech, Language, and Hearing Research, 60*, 2483–2505.

Ward, D. (2017). Stuttering and cluttering: Frameworks for understanding and treatment. Psychology Press. https://doi.org/10.4324/9781315727073

Watkins, K. E., Smith, S. M., Davis, S., & Howell, P. (2008). Structural and functional abnormalities of the motor system in developmental stuttering. *Brain*, 131, 50–59. https://doi.org/10.1093/brain/awm241

Yamasaki, H., LaBar, K. S., & McCarthy, G. (2002). Dissociable prefrontal brain systems for attention and emotion. *Proceedings of the National Academy of Sciences of the United States of America, 99*(17), 11447–11451. https://doi.org/10.1073/pnas.182176499

Module 2

BUILDING SOCIAL PRAGMATIC COMMUNICATION FOR CHILDREN AND TEENS WHO EXPERIENCE ANXIETY IN SPEAKING SITUATIONS

Background Introduction and Theoretical Framework

Module 2 is about conversation and getting better at it. There are 11 practical activities to build conversational skills through interactive games. The focus of this module is for children and teens who have selective mutism and/or who stutter, to improve their social pragmatic communication skills. Often, lack of practice due to anxiety related to selective mutism or stuttering makes conversation more challenging and can impact the individual's core lexicon, expression of main concepts, words per minute, and sharing of information as they converse.

Conversations are an important part of communication. Conversations help people connect in meaningful ways and exchange their thoughts and ideas through more than just words. People who are skilled in conversation have an advantage. They often have friends and acquaintances who enjoy spending time speaking with them. So, what makes someone good at conversation? First, they are good listeners, and they appreciate what someone else has to say. They think about what the other person says, and as they listen, they form their own thoughts, recollections, and images. They wait their turn to speak and add to what the other person said. Each person gives the other time to talk and listens as they speak. Less anxious people tend to have an easier time engaging in conversations. Therefore, it can be beneficial to practice conversational skills.

Asking questions can move conversations forward. Questions introduce new topics, especially open-ended *wh-* questions. Conversations become more meaningful when follow-up questions make the other person think about something of interest. For example, if someone asks, *"What are your favorite classes in school?"* and the response is one word, *"science,"* the conversation could be short-lived. Asking, *"What do you like about science?"* can start a related topic, one that interests both speakers as they learn more about each other. Yes-No questions tend to be conversation stoppers unless the other person says more than *"yes"* or *"no."*

Good conversationalists tend to have various topics they can discuss. They gain their information from doing things, having hobbies, watching TV, reading, spending time getting involved in different experiences, and learning about what is going on in the world. This enhances one's connections in life. But not every moment needs to be filled with talking. Being comfortable listening and showing the other person you are paying attention to what they say is valuable too.

Generally, conversation involves the spontaneous verbal interchange of ideas through connected speech, often related to a variety of topics where people take turns listening and speaking.

According to DeDe and Hoover (2021), conversation is a form of discourse that requires the use of not only pragmatics but also syntax, morphology, phonology, and the cognitive skills of organization, working memory, and theory of mind. This is not an easy process but one that most individuals master. Discourse can take the form of monologues or dialogues. In monologues we tell stories, share procedures to do something, give explanations, and share personal narratives that are important to maintaining relationships. We may also engage in language that has the intent to persuade someone. In dialogues that involve communication with at least two people, we often include conversations, interviews, ordering, and discussions (Cherney et al., 1998).

There are 11 activities and games to develop conversational skills in Module 2 that build on the vocalization work in Module 1. Interactive activities and games in this module are also available for teletherapy through a companion website using an access code found in this manual.

In developing the activities and games in this module, it was important to have the activities build on each other for both responses and initiations, in a hierarchical manner. We begin at the word level while encouraging spontaneous speech output and continue with sentence formulation games. Next, interactive games are used to engage in scripted conversations. We continue with procedural narratives where one person gives directions and another follows them using a barrier-game format. In all activities, the children and teens have a chance to review their accomplishments and learn from their challenges.

Questions, answers, and comments are key to engaging in conversation and important to improving the messages and interactions for children and teens who do not readily speak in situations where speech is expected or who have difficulty with their flow of speech. It is important for children and teens to learn about the power of questions, answers, and comments and how different types give us more or less information. In this module, the child/teen gains confidence as they learn to keep a conversation going. As the communicators take turns speaking and gain new skills, their spontaneity increases as does their ability to engage in conversation and storytelling. Children/teens benefit from opportunities to share information, relate an event, provide comments, agree or disagree, and engage in questioning skills. As this module moves hierarchically forward, the next stage has the child/teen engage in conversational role-plays with photos to gain more experience sharing greetings, showing appreciation, and being able to complain, apologize, request clarification, make an excuse, and ask for help. In the final section, children and teens can use a pre- and post-chat sentence completion questionnaire to compare changes before and after working on conversational topics. Every skill in this module, whether in the paper version or online, includes a game-like activity that children and teens can play.

Children and teens also learn about nonverbal components of conversation. These paralinguistic skills are important to becoming an effective communicator. Although the skills do not involve words, they do influence communicative interactions in a major way. These include the following:

1. *Tone of voice*—People hear expression in one's tone of voice. Even over the phone without video, expression is evident when listening to someone speak. These microexpressions, such as sounding happy, tend to make people pleased. Check out https://www.scienceofpeople.com/ted/
2. *Body language*—Facial expressions, such as smiling or frowning, give clues about how other people feel. Facial expressions are often contagious when

we see genuine emotions from another person. How we move and stand, where we look, and the expressions we portray have an effect on other people. These are part of our conversational toolbox. Practice can help make these skills second nature. Check out https://www.verywellmind.com/understand-body-language-and-facial-expressions-4147228

3. *Hand gestures*—Seeing someone else's hands helps us know their intentions. We feel safer when we see someone's hands because we get a sense about what they are thinking and feeling. Hand gestures when talking help us understand what someone is saying and can even help people explain things with greater ease. Check out https://voices.uchicago.edu/goldinmeadowlab/

These links can be modified based on the facilitator's needs for their individual clients. Some links may become unavailable over time, but related links can be found using a search engine.

Overarching Goals for Module 2

The main goals of Module 2 are to improve three primary areas of social communication. These include (1) using language for different reasons, (2) changing language for the listener or situation, and (3) following rules for conversations and storytelling (American Speech-Language-Hearing Association [ASHA], 2020).

1. Using language for different reasons
   a. Greetings when entering a situation
   b. Farewells when leaving a situation
   c. Thanking to show appreciation
   d. Commenting and complimenting
   e. Apologizing
   f. Requesting clarification and information
   g. Stating a problem and making an excuse
   h. Making a complaint and complaining
   i. Asking for help and offering help
   j. Providing information
2. Changing language for the listener or situation
   a. Assuming different roles
   b. Adjusting interactions with different people
   c. Adjusting interactions in different settings
3. Following rules for conversation and storytelling
   a. Engaging with interest when interacting with others
   b. Listening actively when another person speaks
   c. Giving opinions politely

d. Using intonation/vocal expression in voice
e. Using gestures and body language with facial expression
f. Taking turns speaking using questions, answers, and comments to initiate and respond to a communicative partner
g. Staying on topic, introducing a topic, or changing a topic
h. Telling a story or relating an event about something that happened

The activities in this module intend to help children and teens experience greater ease and comfort communicating. Each activity/game begins with background information and continues with goals, materials, and steps for how to play. Suggestions to enhance treatment for children/teens with selective mutism can be found in Appendix 2–A, and suggestions to enhance treatment for stuttering can be found in Appendix 2–B, both at the end of Module 2. These sections offer strategies and therapeutic suggestions for new learning. The 11 activity titles are as follows:

1. Word Think: The First Word That Comes to Mind
2. Pinpoint: Words to Sentences
3. Actors' Corner: Interactive Scripts
4. Barriers: Following Directions
5. Question Match: Answering Questions
6. More Information Please: Changing Questions
7. See-Saw: Keep the Conversation Going
8. Road Runner: Stay on Topic Track
9. Conversation Wheelhouse: Situational Conversation Skills
10. Conversational Role-Plays: Social Communication
11. Chat Spin: Informal Conversations

Prior to engaging in the activities, the facilitator may want to use The *Social Communication Skills—Pragmatics Checklist* (Goberis et al., 2012) as one of the measures to gather information about the child or teen's social communication skills. This is a valuable tool for analyzing social communication at various levels of verbal output. Ask an adult (parent and/or teacher) to rate the individual's skills at the start of this module by placing a check mark in one of the four columns that best describes how they think the child/teen interacts on each item. These include using complex language, using one to three words, using no words, or identifying that the skill is not present. The measure includes 45 items representing skills about (a) stating needs, (b) giving commands, (c) expressing feelings, (d) interacting with others, (e) asking questions, and (f) sharing information. The checklist can be used as a baseline measure and for monitoring individuals' progress and carryover of skills. The checklist can be found in Table 2–1 and at the following link: https://successforkidswithhearingloss.com/wp-content/uploads/2012/01/PRAGMATICS-CHECKLIST.pdf. Item interpretations of the checklist can be found at https://successforkidswithhearingloss.com/wp-content/uploads/2013/08/Pragmatics-Checklist-Interpretation.pdf. In using this checklist, recall that many social pragmatic communication skills develop early. By 5 years of age, most children have begun to master the six domains of social communication skills on the Pragmatics Checklist.

TABLE 2–1. Social Communication Skills—The Pragmatic Checklist

Child/Teen's Name ______ Date ______ Completed by: ______ **Pragmatic Objectives**	Not Present	Uses NO Words	Uses 1–3 Words	Uses Complex Language
Instrumental—States Needs (I want . . .)				
1. Makes polite requests				
2. Makes choices				
3. Gives description of an object wanted				
4. Expresses a specific personal need				
5. Requests help				
Regulatory—Gives Commands (Do as I tell you....)				
6. Gives directions to play a game				
7. Gives directions to make something				
8. Changes the style of commands or requests depending on whom the child is speaking to and what the child wants				
Personal—Expresses Feelings				
9. Identifies feelings (I'm happy.)				
10. Explains feelings (I'm happy because it's my birthday.)				
11. Provides excuses or reasons				
12. Offers an opinion with support				
13. Complains				
14. Blames others				
15. Provides pertinent information on request (two or three of the following: name, address, phone, birth date)				
Interactional—Me and You . . .				
16. Interacts with others in a polite manner				
17. Uses appropriate social rules such as greetings, farewells, thank you, getting attention				
18. Attends to the speaker				
19. Revises/repairs an incomplete message				
20. Initiates a topic of conversation (doesn't just start talking in the middle of a topic)				
21. Maintains a conversation (able to keep it going)				
22. Ends a conversation (doesn't just walk away)				

continues

TABLE 2–1. *continued*

Pragmatic Objectives	Not Present	Uses NO Words	Uses 1–3 Words	Uses Complex Language
23. Interjects appropriately into an already established conversation with others				
24. Makes apologies or gives explanations of behavior				
25. Requests clarification				
26. States a problem				
27. Criticizes others				
28. Disagrees with others				
29. Compliments others				
30. Makes promises				
Wants Explanations—Tell me Why . . .				
31. Asks questions to get more information				
32. Asks questions to systematically gather information as in "Twenty Questions"				
33. Asks questions because of curiosity				
34. Asks questions to problem-solve (What should I do? How do I know?)				
35. Asks questions to make predictions (What will happen if…?)				
Shares Knowledge & Imaginations—I've got something to tell you . . .				
36. Role-play as/with different characters				
37. Role-plays with props (i.e., banana as phone)				
38. Provides a description of a situation that describes the main events				
39. Correctly re-tells a story that has been told to them				
40. Relates the content of a four- to six-frame picture story using correct events for each frame				
41. Creates an original story with a beginning, several logical events, and an end				
42. Explains the relationship between two objects, actions, or situations				
43. Compares and contrasts qualities of two objects, actions, or situations				
44. Tells a lie				
45. Expresses humor/sarcasm				
Totals				

Activity Game 1: Word Think—The First Word That Comes to Mind

Goals of the Activity

- To say a word spontaneously without lengthy pausing or hesitations

In this activity, the child or teen works to say words with spontaneity, reducing hesitations. This activity is intended to improve listening and speed of processing without concern for a right or wrong response. The two people engaged in this activity are working on initiating and responding by saying words in a dynamic interchange, each taking turns and saying any word that comes to mind. For example, if the facilitator says *car,* the child/teen can say *drive, wheel, tires, road,* or any other word that comes to mind.

Materials

- Word Associations List with 48 common words composed of nouns, verbs, and adjectives (Table 2–2).

Word List for This Activity

See Table 2–2 on page 55. Think of more words!

How to Play

The facilitator says the words, one at a time. It is recommended to cut that page on the dotted lines so each word is separated. Turn the words over and choose one at a time for the activity. Tell the child, *"When you hear a word or read it, say the first word that comes to your mind. Any word is fine. There is no right or wrong answer. You can even make up a new word or a silly word. For example, if I say 'up' you can say 'down' or you can say 'sky' or you can say 'pup' or any word you think of. You can even repeat the word that I said."* Let them know that they should say their word as soon as they can, not to pause too long. Change places with the child/teen. Let them decide if they want to do 12, 24, 36, or 48 words to start during any given session. They can earn points by saying more words. Set up a motivational system to earn rewards.

Suggestions to enhance treatment for children/teens with selective mutism can be found in Appendix 2–A, and suggestions to enhance treatment for stuttering can be found in Appendix 2–B, both at the end of Module 2.

The online version of this activity includes an interactive game.

Activity Game 2: Pinpoint—Words to Sentences

Goals of the Activity

- To say what comes to mind spontaneously
- To take turns speaking
- To formulate sentences on topic

In this activity, the child or teen works on generating simple to complex sentence formulations, following up on what was said previously. Communicating is not just about being able to talk; it is also about what one conveys when they talk. It involves attending to the speaker, making word choices, and engaging in spontaneous sentences to convey a message.

Each of the words used in this activity represents a *noun* (person, place, thing, or idea); a *verb* (words that have action or express a state of being); *adjectives* (words that describe a noun or pronoun); and *adverbs* (words that modify an adjective, verb, or another adverb). To be classified as a sentence, a noun and verb must be used. Sentences between speakers should also be cohesive, in other words, follow a topic or a related topic.

- The child/teen and facilitator can take turns making sentences that connect to form a conversation around a topic.
- Remind the child or teen that they are the *Communicator-in-Chief.*

Materials

- Common Word Lists (Table 2–3)

How to Play

Use the word lists in Table 2–3 for this activity. Tell the child or teen, "*In this activity you will create your own sentences. You can choose any word from the word list with the aim to use four words from the row in your sentence. We will take turns saying a sentence related to what the previous person said. For example, if one person uses the word 'time' and says, 'I enjoy my time watching TV,' the other person can choose the word 'out' from the word list (if it hasn't been used) and say, 'I'm the kind of person who would rather go out.' Take turns with the aim to make up sentences for four words in a row (either top-to-bottom, left-to-right, or diagonally). To win, you can choose a word that will block the other person from getting four in a row.*" To keep score, either copy the 4 × 4 word list and circle your words with different colors or use chips or another identifying marker. Table 2–4 can be used to track the words said in sentences.

Suggestions to enhance treatment for children/teens with selective mutism can be found in Appendix 2–A, and suggestions to enhance treatment for stuttering can be found in Appendix 2–B, both at the end of Module 2.

The online version of this activity includes an interactive game.

TABLE 2–2. Word Associations List

my	more	music	mustard
no	money	pencil	paper
shoe	truck	drink	star
magic	swim	nose	sleep
eat	read	apple	kick
mouth	doctor	candy	light
play	monkey	puppy	fun
long	cake	game	flag
baby	red	ball	see
tiger	nest	milk	TV
farm	glass	ring	drive
throw	happy	girl	home

TABLE 2–3. Common Word Lists

Group 1				
NOUN	time	person	year	way
VERB	be	have	do	any word
ADJECTIVE	good	new	first	last
ADVERB	up	any word	out	just
Group 2				
NOUN	day	thing	any word	world
VERB	get	make	go	know
ADJECTIVE	any word	great	little	own
ADVERB	now	how	then	more
Group 3				
NOUN	life	hand	part	child
VERB	take	see	any word	think
ADJECTIVE	other	any word	right	big
ADVERB	also	here	well	only
Group 4				
NOUN	eye	woman	place	any word
VERB	look	want	give	any word
ADJECTIVE	high	different	small	any word
ADVERB	very	even	back	any word

Source: From *English Club*, J. Essberger, 2020. https://www.englishclub.com/vocabulary/common-words.htm

TABLE 2–4. Scoring Common Words

Noun	Verb	Adjective	Adverb	Player 1				Player 2			
time	be	good	up								
person	have	new	any words								
year	do	first	out								
way	any word	last	just								
day	get	any word	now								
thing	make	great	how								
any word	go	little	then								
world	know	own	more								
life	take	other	also								
hand	see	any word	here								
part	any word	right	well								
child	think	big	only								
eye	look	high	very								
woman	want	different	even								
place	give	small	back								
any word	any word	any word	any word								
Total Points: (One point per word used in sentences)				______				______			

Activity Game 3: Actors' Corner—Interactive Scripts

Goals of the Activity

- To use intonation and vocal expression
- To engage in dialogue with turn-taking and topic maintenance
- To increase communicative interactions with scripted conversation

In this activity, the child or teen works on engaging the communication partner and speaking using interactive scripted conversations. Social communication is important at this age and evolving during the school-age years. Children learn to read body language and facial expressions and understand the meanings behind various vocal intonations to know how someone is feeling. They can tell a story and engage in a conversation with turn-taking and topic maintenance. They display good social conventions and can use language to give their opinion and persuade someone (Russell, 2007).

In the Actors' Corner activity, interactive scripts are provided. The scripts include sentences for two people to read aloud with several sentence completions. To further assist with vocal and facial expression, the facilitator can provide a model and ask the child or teen to imitate how something was said. According to Voncken and Bögels (2008), interactions that include interpersonal skills, such as conversational tasks and role-plays, help the child or teen gain more experience with social performance, thereby reducing social anxiety. Gaining experience with new communication partners through role-plays can help reduce avoidance and improve interactions.

Materials

- Scripted dialogue with short interactive scenarios (Figures 2–1 to 2–4)
- For children who need additional help reading, read the script or say the sentences for them to repeat

The Scripts

Title: Discovery of the Twig Boat (Figure 2–1)

This script is about two friends watching at the edge of the river, watching what looks like a rowboat floating toward them. Decide on names you would like to use for this role-play script and who is going first. Try to use expression when speaking, if appropriate.

Name 1—*Look at that in the water. It looks like a rowboat.*

Name 2—*It really does.*

Name 1—*Yeah. It looks like an old rowboat.*

Name 2—*When it gets closer what should we do?*

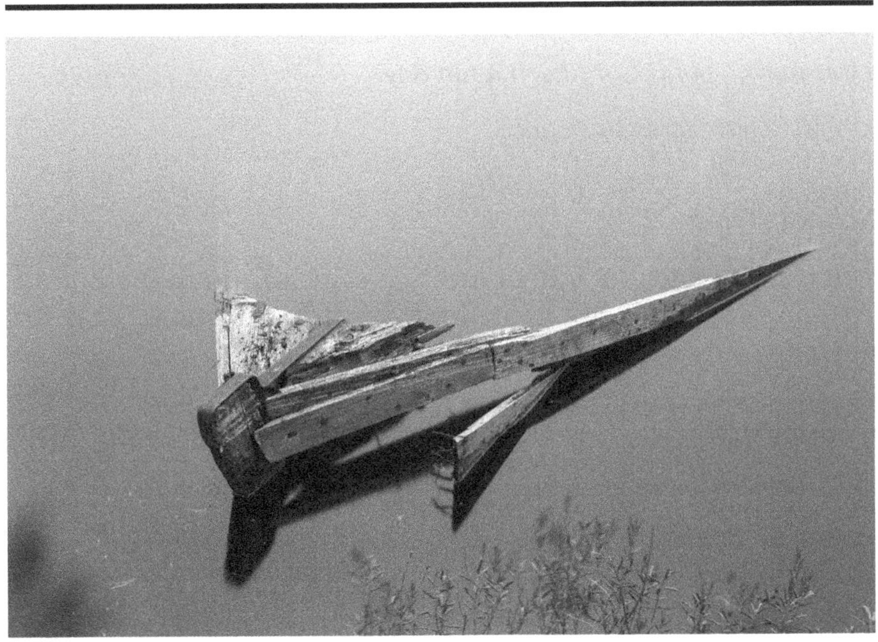

FIGURE 2–1. Twig boat.

Name 1—*Let's go down to the edge of the river. We'll get closer to see it.*

Name 2—*It's coming closer, and it looks kind of small.*

Name 1—*You're right. It doesn't seem to be that good at all. What is it?*

Name 2—*I don't know. It doesn't have any sails either.*

Name 1—*I think it's just a little broken rowboat now that it's getting closer.*

Name 2—*You're right. It's just a rowboat.*

Name 1—*Maybe there is something cool inside it. Maybe we can get in it.*

Name 2—*Great idea! We could still have some fun.*

Name 1—*Let's go before anyone else gets to it.*

Name 2—*Oh no, I can't believe this. Now that we're up close, it's just a bunch of twigs that were tied together.*

Name 1—*There's nothing we can do with this now. I am so disappointed.*

Name 2—*Me too. We waited here all this time and all we see is a bunch of twigs.*

Name 1—*Do you have any other good ideas? I'm afraid to ask!*

Name 2—*Well, you know, we could take the twigs back home and make something with them.*

Name 1—*If we put holes in the ends of each twig and line them up from shortest at the top to longest at the bottom, we can use a rope to tie them together, like a Christmas tree.*

Name 2—*That's a really good idea. Do you have the tools we need like a drill and rope?*

Name 1—*I think so, and someone at my house can help us if we need it.*

Name 2—*This is going to be a great project and maybe even a good gift for someone.*

Name 1—*So this worked out OK. It's been a fun day!*

Name 2—*Yeah, we'll have to do this again.*

Title: New at School (Figure 2–2)

This script is about a new student at school meeting a friend. Fill in the blanks with your own words. Decide on names you would like to use for this script and who is going first. Remember to use expression in your voice as appropriate.

Name 1—*Hi. My name is ____________. Are you new here at school?*

Name 2—*Yeah. My name is ____________. I just started here.*

Name 1—*So what do you think of this place?*

Name 2—*It's OK. Kinda strange since I don't know anyone really.*

Name 1—*I can show you around, and I'll introduce you to some of my friends.*

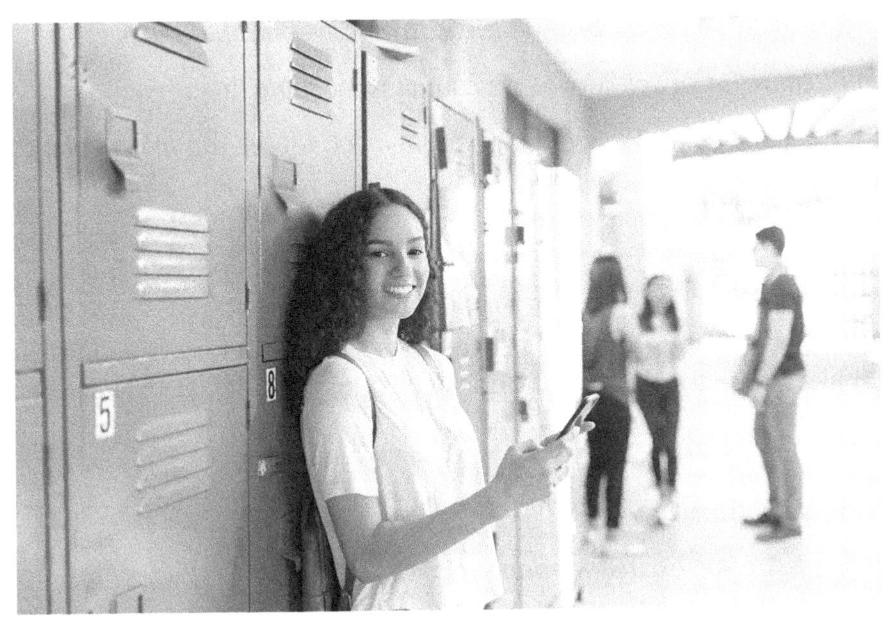

FIGURE 2–2. New at school.

Name 2—*That sounds good.*

Name 1—*Who's your homeroom teacher?*

Name 2—*It's ____________. Who's yours?*

Name 1—*Mine is ____________. She's OK, but I really don't spend a lot of time in homeroom.*

Name 2—*What do you like to do here at school? Are you in any clubs?*

Name 1—*I play field hockey and I like it. I'm pretty good at it. The coach is OK.*

Name 2—*I never played field hockey, but I did run track at my old school.*

Name 1—*That's cool. You can come to one of my practices and watch. Maybe you could join since you ran track.*

Name 2—*I would like that. When is your next practice or game?*

Name 1—*It's Friday. Yeah. Come if you can.*

Name 2—*What time do you play and where?*

Name 1—*We play in the field out back of the school. It's at 3:00. Definitely come. It'll be fun. I'll introduce you to the coach.*

Name 2—*OK. I'll be there. I just have to let my parents know I'll be late coming back from school. They'll have to pick me up.*

Name 1—*I can have my mom drop you off. Where do you live?*

Name 2—*I live in the new houses on Jackson St. I'm at 24 Jackson St.*

Name 1—*I know exactly where that is! My friend Taylor lives on that block.*

Name 2—*I don't know Taylor yet. Maybe we can all meet some time.*

Name 1—*That would be great. Well, glad we got to meet. I'll see you at school and at field hockey.*

Name 2—*Yeah, thanks! See ya.*

Title: Dance Class (Figure 2–3)

This script is about a person at dance class meeting a friend before the class starts. Decide on names you would like to use for this script and who is going first. Use expression if needed.

Name 1—*Hi. How are you?*

Name 2—*Hi. I'm good. How are you?*

Name 1—*I'm good. Are you excited for dance class?*

Name 2—*Yeah! This is my favorite class.*

Name 1—*Me too.*

Name 2—*I hope we do lyrical today.*

Name 1—*I like how we do lyrical on Tuesdays and tap and ballet on Mondays.*

Name 2—*I like how we do jazz on Wednesdays too.*

Name 1—*What are you doing the 2 weeks we're off?*

Name 2—*I'm relaxing! What about you?*

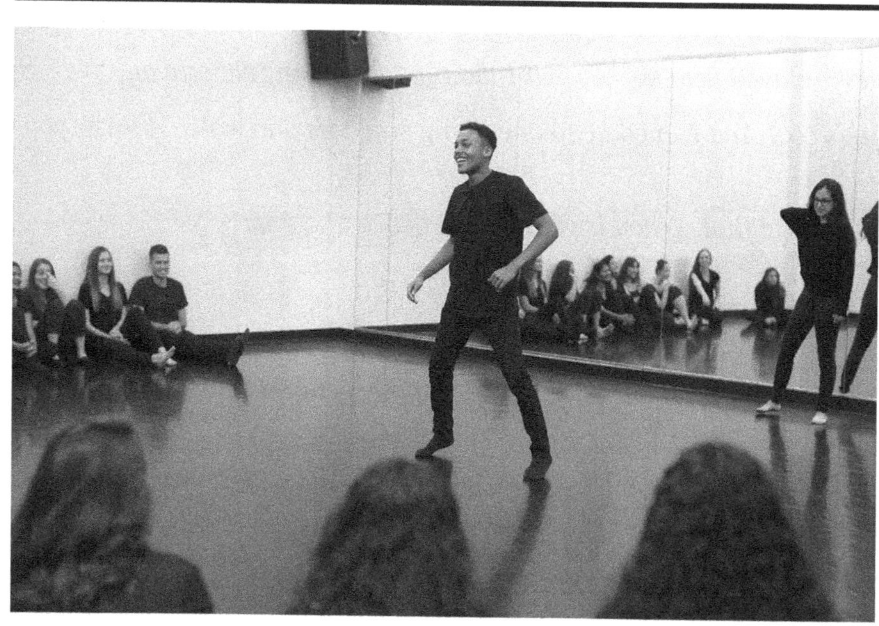

FIGURE 2–3. Dance class.

Name 1—*I'm relaxing too. I'm going to catch up on some shows.*

Name 2—*What shows do you like?*

Name 1—*I like* ___________.

Name 2—*I like that too. I'm up to season 3. How much have you watched?*

Name 1—*I'm up to season 2.*

Name 2—*I liked season 2 a lot.*

Name 1—*I like it too. Don't tell me what happens.*

Name 2—*I won't.*

Name 1—*I think* ___________ *are going to* ___________ *in the show.*

Name 2—*I'm not telling because I don't wanna spoil it for you.*

Name 1—*Thank you!*

Name 2—*You're welcome.*

Name 1—*We better get into dance now.*

Name 2—*Yeah!*

Title: The Birthday (Figure 2–4)

This script is about a person asking someone in the family or a friend about what gift they would like for their birthday. Decide on names you would like to use for this script and who is going first. Fill in the blanks. Use expression if needed.

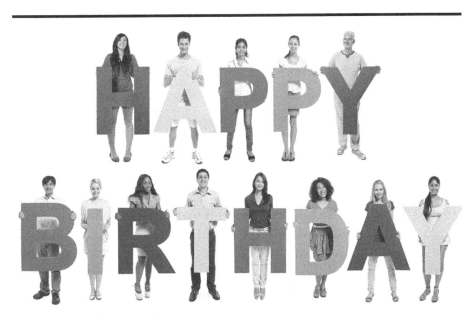

FIGURE 2–4. The birthday.

Name 1—*Have you thought about what you want for a birthday gift?*

Name 2—*Yeah, I really want* ___________.

Name 1—*Wow, that's an interesting gift!*

Name 2—*I know and* ___________.

Name 1—*I agree. I just don't know if* ___________.

Name 2—*If I can't get that what do you think about* ___________?

Name 1—*That's OK. Let me look into it.*

Name 2—*I would like either one so* ___________.

Name 1—*You know I want you to have a good present.*

Name 2—*Thanks. What about your birthday?*

Name 1—*What about it? It's not until* ___________.

Name 2—*I'll remember to get you something.*

Name 1—*I know you will. You're very* ___________.

Name 2—*Maybe we could go somewhere too.*

Name 1—*Where would you like to go?*

Name 2—*I would like to go* ___________.

Name 1—*I'm not sure about going there because* ___________.

Name 2—*Let's think about other places to go.*

Name 1—*How about if we go* ___________.

Name 2—*That's a good idea. I would like that because* ___________.

Name 1—*Great, and we can* ___________.

Name 2—*That's a good idea. I have to get going, but I'm glad we had a chance to talk.*

Name 1—*Me too.*

Name 2—*See you later.*

How to Play

Use the scripts as a guide. Take turns reading the parts aloud. Add expression to voice as appropriate. Each person should fill in the blanks with their own thoughts. The child/teen may imitate the facilitator to practice vocal expressions. At the end of each script, talk about the experience. Check out the link https://www.dramanotebook.com/plays-for-kids/ for more scripts. There are original royalty-free scripts (although there is a fee for joining) for elementary, middle, and high school students on the website. These include short plays, one-act plays, and full scripts. There are plays from which to choose that include a few or many actors. The players can assume one or more roles. Changing voices for different characters can add an element of fun.

Suggestions to enhance treatment for children/teens with selective mutism can be found in Appendix 2–A, and suggestions to enhance treatment for stuttering can be found in Appendix 2–B, both at the end of Module 2.

The online version of this activity includes an interactive game.

Activity Game 4: Barriers—Following Directions

Goals of the Activity

- To increase listening skills
- To increase direction-giving skills
- To request clarification
- To help reduce possible perfectionistic tendencies

In this activity, the child or teen works on following instructions, giving verbal directions, and asking questions for clarification if anything is not clear. Children and teens with social communication anxiety often experience fear and anticipate negative social interactions. In a study by Vassilopoulos and Banerjee (2010), even when a social event went well, students worried about the next event not going as well and thought that if they did well previously, people would expect more from them the next time. Pressure to perform well all the time can put a great burden on anyone. The activities to follow require the child/teen to engage in a social performance challenge using drawing. The child or teen is encouraged to ask for clarification whenever directions are unclear to them. They are given spoken instructions to draw an image.

When completed, they review their drawing and compare it with the sample (Figures 2–5 through 2–7). The facilitator can discuss feelings associated with making a perceived mistake. By pointing out information that was unclear in the instructions, cognitive restructuring can help the child or teen better cope with any perceived imperfection.

Materials

- Drawing instructions
- Paper, pencil, pen, or markers

How to Play

Place a paper (regular 8½ × 11 is best) on a steady surface and get a pencil, pen, or markers to draw. Listen to the instructions given by the other person, one at a time, and follow them. If anything is unclear or the child/teen needs to hear the instructions again, tell them to ask for more information or for the other person to repeat what was said. After all the instructions are given, each will share their drawings to see if they match. The instructions are spoken at first. They can be read by the direction-follower too, before sharing each other's drawings, if desired. Take turns giving new instructions for additional drawings.

The Drawings

Drawing 1

Remind the child/teen to ask a question for clarification or repetition if they are not sure what to do.

1. *Draw a square in the center of the paper.*
2. *Draw a circle inside the square.*
3. *Draw an X inside the circle.*
4. *Draw a zig-zag line outside each side of the square.*

Let's review.

- *How do you think you did with following my directions?*
- *What would you think if your drawing doesn't turn out like the one I am going to show you?*
- *You know, my directions weren't perfect. I could have added more descriptions. For example, when I said to draw a zig-zag line outside each side of the square, I didn't say what direction to draw the lines, did I?*
- *Now, look at your drawing compared to the sample.*
- *What do you think?*
- *No one ever gets the instructions perfect. My directions left things to the imagination. It's OK if you did yours differently.*
- *Even if you didn't listen to everything I said or didn't follow the directions perfectly and your drawing looks different than mine, can you be OK with that?*

Show the sample drawing after you see the child/teen's drawing (Figure 2–5). Discuss them. Point out that no one is expecting perfection and that some directions may not have been clear or even given. It is fine to redo it again after seeing the sample drawing. Revision is a good teaching tool.

Drawing 2

Remind the child/teen to ask for clarification/repetition if they are not sure what to do.

1. *Draw a big circle in the center of the paper.*
2. *Draw a triangle pointing upward with the bottom part touching the top of the circle.*
3. *Draw a small triangle in the middle of the big circle.*
4. *Draw two small circles, slightly above and to each side of that small triangle.*
5. *Draw one dot inside each small circle.*
6. *Draw a curve below the small triangle.*
7. *Draw a line from the bottom center of the big circle to the bottom of the paper.*

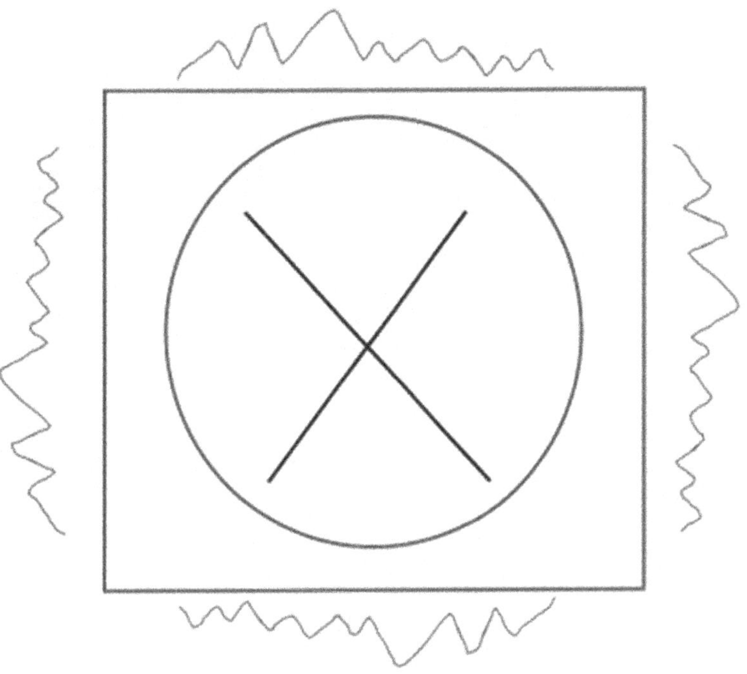

FIGURE 2–5. Sample Drawing 1—X in box.

8. *Draw another long line next to the one you just drew so you have a double line.*
9. *Draw two small half circles, one on each side of the big circle.*
10. *Draw one line going across the middle of the bottom two long lines.*
11. *Draw two circles, one on the end of each side of the line going across.*
12. *Draw a star at the top of the big triangle.*

Let's review.

- *How do you think you did with following my directions?*
- *What would you think if your drawing doesn't turn out like the one I am going to show you?*
- *You know, my directions weren't perfect. I could have added more descriptions. For example, when I said to draw a curve below the small triangle, I didn't say what kind of curve to draw, did I?*
- *Look at your drawing compared to the sample* (Figure 2–6).
- *What do you think?*
- *No one ever gets the instructions perfect. My directions left things to the imagination. It's OK if you did yours differently.*
- *Even if you didn't listen to everything I said or didn't follow the directions perfectly and your drawing looks different than mine, can you be OK with that?*

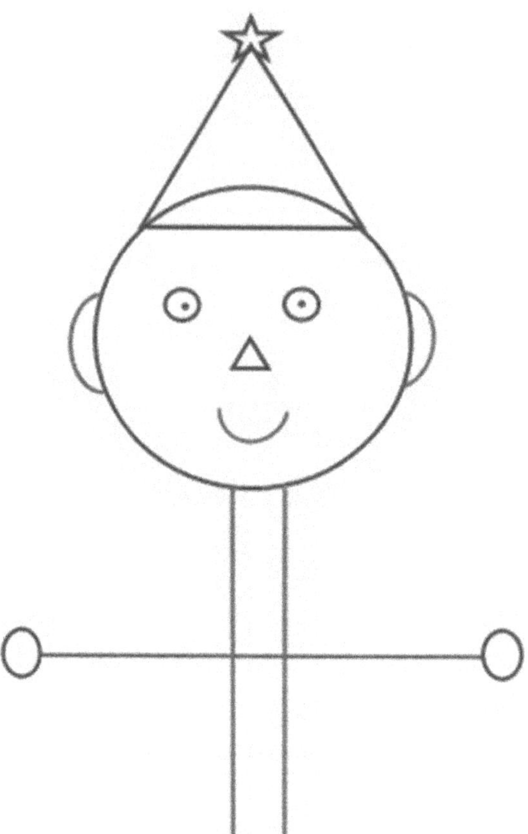

FIGURE 2–6. Sample Drawing 2—Face with hat.

Drawing 3—Circle and Four Faces

Remind the child/teen to ask for clarification/repetition if they are not sure what to do.

1. *Draw four circles, one in each corner of the paper.*
2. *Draw one big circle in the center of the paper.*
3. *Draw a line connecting each corner circle to the big center circle.*
4. *Draw a bigger circle around the circle in the center of the paper.*
5. *Draw four arrows, one inside each space between the center circle lines.*
6. *Draw a heart inside the big center circle.*
7. *Using scribbles, shade in the heart with your pencil, pen, or marker.*
8. *Draw scribbles on the top of each of the four corner circles.*
9. *Draw a happy face inside the top left corner circle.*
10. *Draw a sad face inside the top right corner circle.*
11. *Draw a mad/angry face inside the bottom left corner circle.*
12. *Draw a surprised face inside the bottom right corner circle.*

Let's review.

- *How do you think you did with following my directions?*
- *What would you think if your drawing doesn't turn out like the one I am going to show you?*
- *You know, my directions weren't perfect. I could have added more descriptions. For example, when I said to draw four arrows, one inside each space between the center circle lines, I didn't say which way to draw the arrows, did I?*
- *Look at your drawing compared to the sample* (Figure 2–7).
- *What do you think?*
- *No one ever gets the instructions perfect. My directions left things to the imagination. It's OK if you did yours differently.*
- *Even if you didn't listen to everything I said or didn't follow the directions perfectly and your drawing looks different than mine, are you OK with that?*

Your Turn to Give Instructions

Tell the child or teen to give the directions. *"Tell me what shapes or objects to draw and where to place them on the page. Make up anything you like. As you give me the directions, draw each one yourself on your own paper and don't let me see it (use a barrier of anything to block each other's views of drawings) until we are finished. When you have given me about five or more instructions, we can check to see if my drawing matches yours. You can choose circles, squares, triangles, rectangles, other shapes, lines, letters, or any objects you want us to draw."*

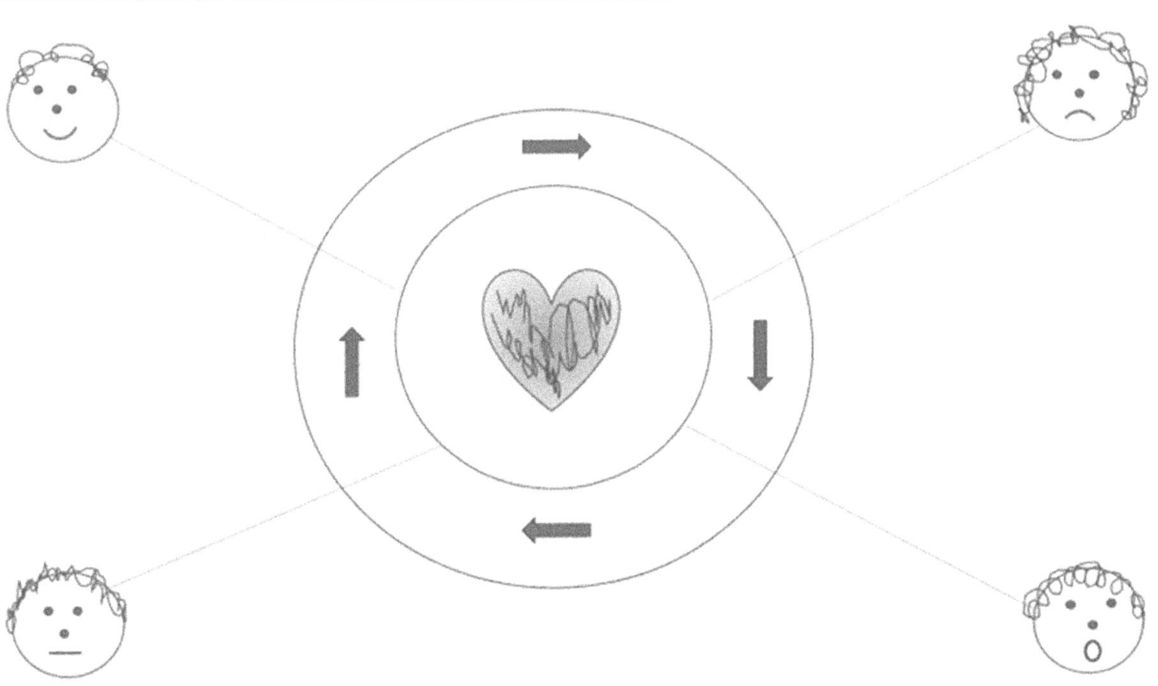

FIGURE 2–7. Sample Drawing 3—Circle with four faces.

Suggestions to enhance treatment for children/teens with selective mutism can be found in Appendix 2–A, and suggestions to enhance treatment for stuttering can be found in Appendix 2–B, both at the end of Module 2.

The online version of this activity includes an interactive game.

Activity Game 5: Question Match—Answering Questions

Goals of the Activity

- To provide or request information (yes-no and *wh-* questions)
- To engage in turn-taking and question-answer routines
- To give sufficient information for listener comprehension and interaction

In this activity, the child or teen works on asking and answering questions and giving reasons for their responses. Asking and answering questions are key to communication and forming relationships. Questions are part of initiating conversations ("How are you?" "What's new?") or leaving conversations ("Will I see you later?" "When can we meet again?"). People learn through questioning. They ask for help, request clarification, and ask for information. This activity lends itself to practicing many yes-no and *wh-* questions with modeling. Children usually enjoy thinking about what to say to answer questions. This can improve their ability to engage in conversations and discussions (Ukrainetz, 2015).

Materials

- Yes-No Question cards (Table 2–5)
- *Wh-* Question cards (Table 2–6)
- Variety Question cards (Table 2–7)
- Number cards (Table 2–8)

Yes-No Questions

Why do you think people ask questions?

What seems to be the difference between yes-no questions and *wh-* questions?

To follow up, share some acceptable photos of people in different places using your phone. Ask the child/teen to ask you questions about the photo (who the people are, where they were at the time, and/or what was happening) to learn more. Offer comments related to the photo. For children who need additional help answering different types of open-ended *wh-* questions (who, what, where, when, how, and why), check out free printable *wh-* questions at https://www.speechtherapystore.com/wh-questions-worksheets/

TABLE 2–5. Yes or No Question Cards

Do you like to play a sport?	Have you decided what you would like to do for a job when you are finished school or college?	Is there a video game you like to play?
Does anyone in your class seem to get special attention from the teacher?	Do you have a favorite TV show?	Can you play a musical instrument?
Are you having a good time?	Is your teacher giving a lot of homework?	Are you going to have a vacation this year?
Does anyone in your family like to eat ice cream?	Can you find something to do when you feel bored?	Have you gone any place other than home or school in the past month?

TABLE 2–6. Wh- Question Cards

Who do you like to get together with?	When do you think people should be able to drive a car?	What would you like to buy if you had as much money as you want?
How do you get your parent(s) to give you what you want?	Why do you think kids are taught to say please and thank you?	Who is someone you want to be friends with?
Where do you like to eat out?	When is your birthday?	How do you feel when there is a thunderstorm?
Why should children go to school?	Where do you like to go to have a good time?	What are two wishes you would like to come true?

TABLE 2–7. Variety Question Cards

To answer these questions, add the word <u>*because*</u> to the end of the sentence to add a reason, if appropriate.

Who do you like to spend time with? Why do you choose that person?	Do you like going to school or staying home more? Why is that?	Where would you like to live if you could move anywhere? Why?
How do you feel about having visitors to your house? What makes you feel that way?	What is one of your favorite memories from the time you were younger?	When do you prefer to do your homework? Why do you choose that?
What are some of your favorite things to do?	Do you think this activity is good for practicing conversation?	What makes you feel happy?
What type of TV shows or movies do you like best? Why is that your favorite?	Are you an early day person or a late-night person? How do you know?	What makes you feel sad?

TABLE 2–8. Number Cards

1	5	9
2	6	10
3	7	11
4	8	12

How to Play

Cut the question squares from a selected table into 12 cards. Turn them over so the writing is face down. Shuffle the cards around. On top of each question card place a number card from 1 to 12.

Players can also use two dice to spin to determine which card (number 1 to 12) to read and answer. Otherwise, choose any number or place the separated cards in a bag and choose one at a time. Score a point for each question asked and each answer given. Take turns speaking as you ask and answer questions to learn more about another person.

For a greater challenge, a memory game can be played with the question cards. Each yes-no question type (do, does, is, are, can, and have) has two different questions.

- Have the child/teen choose a number from 1 to 12 and read the question and answer it.
- Then choose another number and see if the question words matched.
- If it matches (e.g., two questions begin with "Do"), read those questions and answer them.
- If the two question types do not match, turn them both back over but remember where they are for the next turn.
- Take turns until all the matching question cards are found!

The same memory game can be played for the *wh-* question cards (who what, where, when, how, and why). There are two cards for each *wh-* question type.

Suggestions to enhance treatment for children/teens with selective mutism can be found in Appendix 2–A, and suggestions to enhance treatment for stuttering can be found in Appendix 2–B, both at the end of Module 2.

The online version of this activity includes an interactive game.

Activity Game 6: More Information Please—Changing Questions

Goals of the Activity

- To ask questions with intonation and vocal expression
- To listen when another person speaks
- To take turns asking and answering questions
- To make a follow-up comment after the other person answers the question

In this activity, the child or teen works on changing yes-no questions to *wh-* questions to learn more about someone else. Questions, answers, follow-up questions, and comments are used in communication every day. It is one of the first ways people learn about other people.

Practicing question-asking is valuable to gather information, learn about new things, get permission, and request clarification when things are unclear. It is one of the main ways we get to know other people and form relationships. For many children or teens with social communication difficulties, these skills are challenging. Questions and answers involve turn-taking during conversational exchanges. Children and teens can use language to ask questions, respond to those of others, and expand their social participation. This activity helps children engage in two-way communication and shows them how changing a question from a yes-no format into a *wh-* format offers them the opportunity to gather more information about a topic, enriching their learning (Laugeson, 2017).

Materials

- Yes-No and *Wh-* Extension Questions
- Table 2–9, Yes-No and *Wh-* Extension Questions

How to Play

Yes-No questions give limited information. Sometimes a person will answer a yes-no question and then add more information. For example, if asked, "Do you have pets?" the person can say, "Yes" or nod their head and then give more details by saying, "Yes, I have a ______" (and talk about their pets).

The task in this activity is to change a yes-no question to a *wh-* question (who, what, where, when, why, or how) to get more information the first time. "Do you have pets?" can be changed to, "What pets do you have or what pets do you want?" That way, the other person knows how to answer your question to give more information. It can be appropriate to start with a yes-no question if the other person is not well known but then to follow up with the *wh-* question if they seem interested in talking but did not add more information on their own.

- Cut the yes-no question sentences into strips, fold them in half, and put them in a bag or other container to pick one when it is your turn.
- As an alternative, you can use the spinning wheel link at https://wheelofnames.com/# and insert numbers on the wheel from 1 to 18 to account for each sentence strip. To do so, simply erase the names in the note box and replace with one number on each line. Press the enter key after each number is entered. When done, put your cursor on the wheel and click it to spin. It will stop at a number.
- Answer with "yes" or "no" on the paper strips marked with "a" (1a) and then attempt to guess the *wh-* question that can give more information on the paper strips marked with "b" (1b).
- Take turns asking each other the same *wh-* questions to learn more about the other person.
- Score a point for each *wh-* question answered.

Suggestions to enhance treatment for children/teens with selective mutism can be found in Appendix 2–A, and suggestions to enhance treatment for stuttering can be found in Appendix 2–B, both at the end of Module 2.

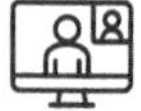

The online version of this activity includes an interactive game.

TABLE 2–9. Yes-No and Wh- Extension Questions

Item Number	Yes-No Questions	Changed to *Wh*- Question
1	1a—Do you have pets?	1b—What pets do you have or want?
2	2a—Do you have any sisters or brothers?	2b—How many sisters or brothers do you have?
3	3a—Do you like music?	3b—What music do you like?
4	4a—Do you like to play video games?	4b—What video games do you like to play?
5	5a—Do you have a favorite TV show?	5b—What is your favorite TV show?
6	6a—Do you know the type of car you want to drive?	6b—What type of car would you like to drive?
7	7a—Do you play a musical instrument?	7b—What musical instrument do you play or want to play?
8	8a—Are there certain types of people you like as friends?	8b—What types of people do you like as friends?
9	9a—Did you go out for your birthday?	9b—Where did you go for your birthday?
10	10a—Do you use social media?	10b—What do you use social media for?
11	11a—Do you have a favorite dessert?	11b—What is your favorite dessert?
12	12a—Do you stay up late on the weekend?	12b—How late do you stay up on the weekend?
13	13a—Do you have a favorite place to eat out?	13b—Where do you like to go to eat out?
14	14a—Do you go to sleep early?	14b—When do you go to sleep at night?
15	15a—Do you have someone special you like to spend time with?	15b—Who do you like to spend time with?
16	16a—Do you know why you get together with relatives?	16b—Why do you get together with relatives?
17	17a—Do you know who is president of the United States?	17b—Who is president of the United States?
18	18a—Is this game going okay foryou?	18b—How is this game going for you?

Activity Game 7: See-Saw—Keep the Conversation Going

Goals of the Activity

- To engage in turn-taking during a conversation
- To ask/answer yes-no questions (is, are, do, does, will, was, were, can, has, have, etc.) and *wh-* questions (who, what, where, when, why, how)
- To make comments during a conversation (state an opinion or feeling, agree or disagree, provide information or instructions, state an intent, provide clarification, make a prediction, provide a reason, and offer a suggestion, etc.), based on communicative acts (Devitt & Hanley, 2003).

In this activity, the child or teen works on turn-taking to build conversations. Turn-taking is essential to having a conversation and building relationships and friendships. Turn-taking also requires initiating and responding. According to Voncken and Bögels (2008), conversations require more communicative skills than giving a speech or presentation. Conversational interactions are spontaneous and unplanned. Speakers and listeners must pay attention to comprehend what was said and gather their own thoughts and experiences to express themselves without a script.

For individuals with social pragmatic communication deficits, anxiety can make sharing information and commenting on what others say more difficult. However, doing so is an important aspect for developing friendships (Altman & Taylor, 1973). It is important to gain experience conversing about topics that are meaningful to the child or teen and their communication partners. More practice often leads to greater comfort and reduced anxiety.

Materials

- Table 2–10, Icons for Conversation
- The labeled paper squares are to be copied and cut so that each person has at least eight of each conversational icon.
- Table 2–11, Sheet of Icons for Conversational Turn-Taking

How to Play

1. Think of a topic that interests you and your speaking partner. If you are not sure, ask your speaking partner to write down a few of their favorite topics and choose one from the list.

TABLE 2–10. Backgrounds and Abbreviations / Icons for Conversation

Yes-No Questions	*Wh-* Questions	Answer	Comment
Y-N?	**Wh?**	**Ans**	**Com**

2. Consider a topic from the following list. Take turns initiating the topic.

   Some Topics to Consider for Conversation:

   - Where would you like to go on vacation, and why do you choose that place?
   - Who is a good friend of yours, and why do you like that person?
   - If you could set up the perfect day, what would you do?
   - If you could be any animal, which one would you choose and why?
   - If you could live in a place with a specific type of weather, what weather would you choose and why?
   - What would you like to do when you are a grown-up, and why do you choose that?
   - What is your favorite movie, TV show, or game to play, and what is good about it?
   - What is a good memory you have in your life?
   - Describe what you do during a regular day.
   - If you had three wishes, what would they be?

3. Begin the conversation by asking a question or making a comment.

Each time someone says something, they must identify it as either a Y-N Question, Wh-Question, Answer, or Comment by choosing the symbol for that response (Figure 2–8). Following is a short sample conversation between two people. The conversation that follows is shown with icons in Figure 2–9.

Me—*Will you answer a question for me? I am doing an interview project, and I have to ask five people this question.* (This included a Yes-No Question then a Comment)

You—*Sure, ask me.* (Answer)

Me—*If you could be any animal, what animal would you want to be?* (Wh- Question)

You—*I would be a bird, probably an eagle.* (Answer)

Me—*Why would you want to be an eagle?* (Wh- Question)

You—*I would like to fly.* (Answer)

Me—*I think eagles are amazing birds.* (Comment)

You—*Me too.* (Comment)

Me—*Do you like small birds?* (Yes-No Question)

You—*I just like how they chirp. What do you like?* (Comment then Wh- question)

Continue with your conversation. Use a table or large space to place the icon squares you select (Figure 2–9).

What icons go with each sentence? Now choose the icons that go with the sentences, place them to the right of the sentence, and continue with the conversation, adding icons from left to right on the lines in the following sentences. Here is the conversation.

Me—*I know you like to dance.* ________ *How long have you been a dancer?* ________

You—*I have been a dancer for 9 years.* ________

Me—*That's awesome.* ________ *I wish I could dance.* ________

You—*Do you want to learn how to dance?* ________

Me—*I do.* ________ *I can dance a little, but I don't think I'm really good at dancing.* ________ *How did you learn?* ________

You—*I learned by taking dance classes at a studio.* ________

Me—*What kind of dancing do you do?* ________

You—*I do tap, ballet, jazz, lyrical, and competitive dancing.* ________ *What are your hobbies?* ________

Me—*That's a great question.* ________ *I like to read.* ________ *Do you have a hobby?* ________

You—*I like to spend time with my friends and family and go places.* ________

Continue with your conversation. Use the icons to display your turn-taking dialogue. Use a table or large space to place each icon, from left to right, to match your sentences.

Me—

____

You—

____

4. Each person should try to use all four icons and put down as many as possible. The more icons used, the better the conversational turn-taking. After a few trials, you can set a timer for 3 to 5 minutes and see how many icons were used in your conversation.

Let's review.

- Was that activity easy or difficult?
- Did you learn anything new?
- What did you learn that is worth remembering?
- What topics are your favorite to discuss or talk about?

Suggestions to enhance treatment for children/teens with selective mutism can be found in Appendix 2–A, and suggestions to enhance treatment for stuttering can be found in Appendix 2–B, both at the end of Module 2.

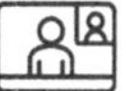

The online version of this activity includes an interactive game.

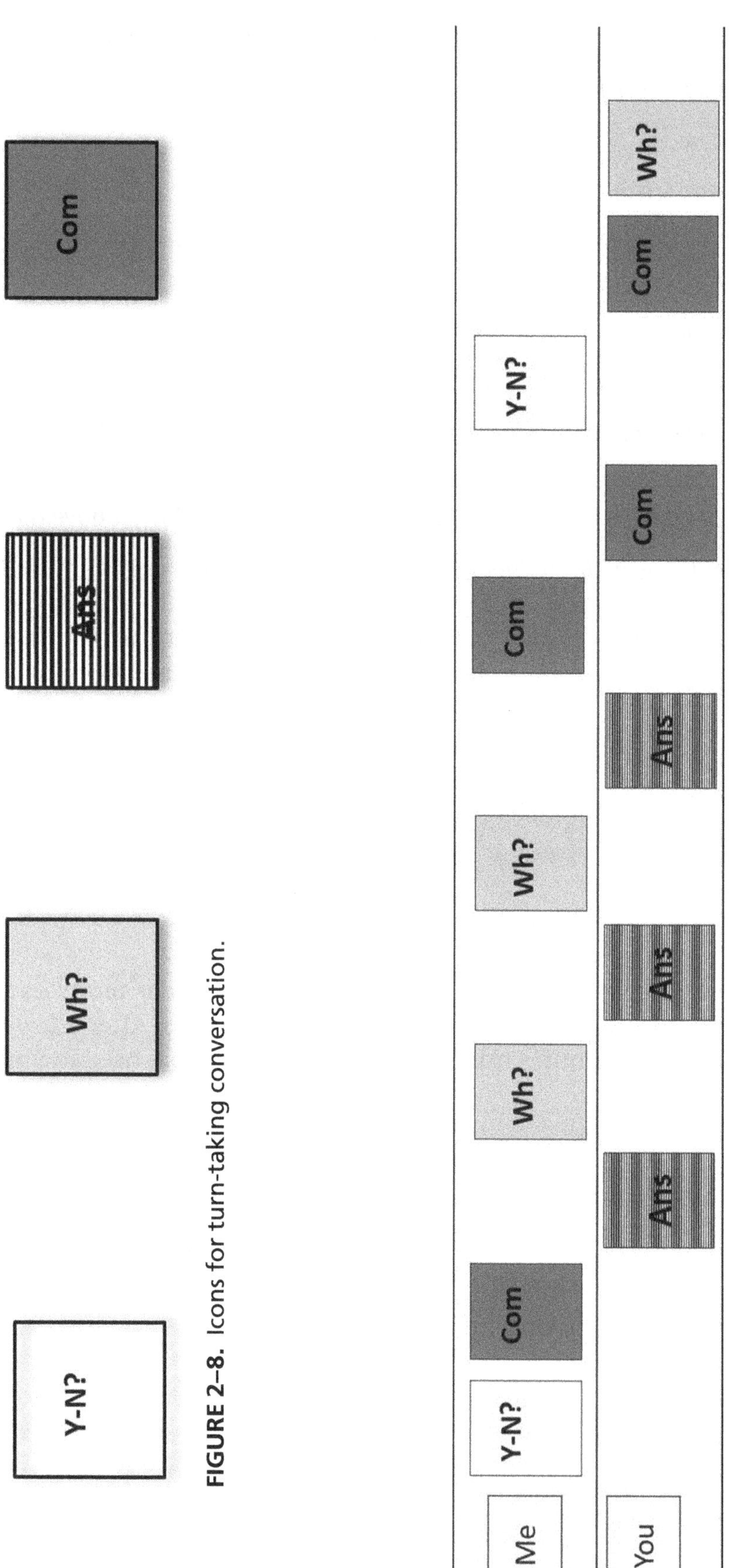

FIGURE 2–8. Icons for turn-taking conversation.

FIGURE 2–9. Icons on lines for conversation.

TABLE 2–11. Sheet of Icons for Conversational Turn-Taking

Icons for Player 1

Y-N?	Wh?	Ans	Com
Y-N?	Wh?	Ans	Com
Y-N?	Wh?	Ans	Com
Y-N?	Wh?	Ans	Com
Y-N?	Wh?	Ans	Com
Y-N?	Wh?	Ans	Com
Y-N?	Wh?	Ans	Com
Y-N?	Wh?	Ans	Com

Icons for Player 2

Y-N?	Wh?	Ans	Com
Y-N?	Wh?	Ans	Com
Y-N?	Wh?	Ans	Com
Y-N?	Wh?	Ans	Com
Y-N?	Wh?	Ans	Com
Y-N?	Wh?	Ans	Com
Y-N?	Wh?	Ans	Com
Y-N?	Wh?	Ans	Com

Activity Game 8: Road Runner—Staying on Topic Track

Goals of the Activity

- To maintain a topic or related topics
- To stay focused and give information for listener comprehension and interaction
- Engage in a two-way conversation and take turns speaking

In this activity, the child or teen works on topic maintenance and turn-taking during conversations. Topic maintenance is important to keeping a conversation going. It requires listening and paying attention to what the conversational partner says. As the person is talking, the listener should imagine a scene or situation that corresponds to what the speaker is saying. Afterward, the other person takes a turn to relate something from their experiences or thoughts that are on the same topic or a related topic.

Conversation assumes turn-taking as people speak to each other. If one person asks the questions and the other person answers with a brief response without any follow-up, the conversation usually ends. On the other hand, if one person monopolizes the conversation, the other person may get tired of just listening. On average, speakers should keep their turn to a maximum of five sentences and then the other person should have a turn to speak, unless telling a story or engaged in a monologue. Pausing for a few seconds usually signals the end of someone's turn and an opportunity for the other person to say something. Facial expressions, intonation, and attending to the speaker are all part of keeping another person engaged and interested in what is being said. As summarized by Michelle Garcia Winner (2007), successful communication involves four primary steps: (1) thinking about the other person, (2) establishing a physical presence so they know you would like to communicate with them, (3) using eye contact to look toward someone prior to speaking to let them know you would like to speak with them, and (4) using language to communicate.

Materials

- Marking utensils (any pencils, pens, markers, crayons, etc.)
- Road map (as shown in Figure 2–11) to copy and write on
- Two markers for turn-taking (Figure 2–10)
- Staying on topic track (Figure 2–11)

How to Play

- There are two drivers (or speakers) whose goal it is to try to stay out of the center of the rectangular frame.
- Once a speaker goes off topic or does not respond (stays silent), that speaker must move (or draw) their arrow to the next inner frame toward the center.
- Make a copy of the track or draw a new one on a clean sheet of paper.

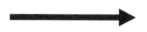

Staying on Topic or related topic – move straight

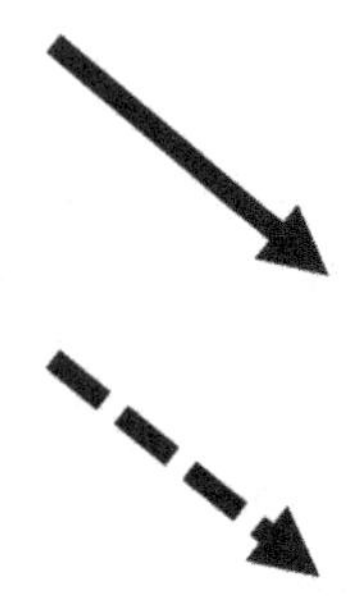

Going off topic or staying silent – move inward to an inner portion of the track

FIGURE 2–10. Two markings for turn-taking.

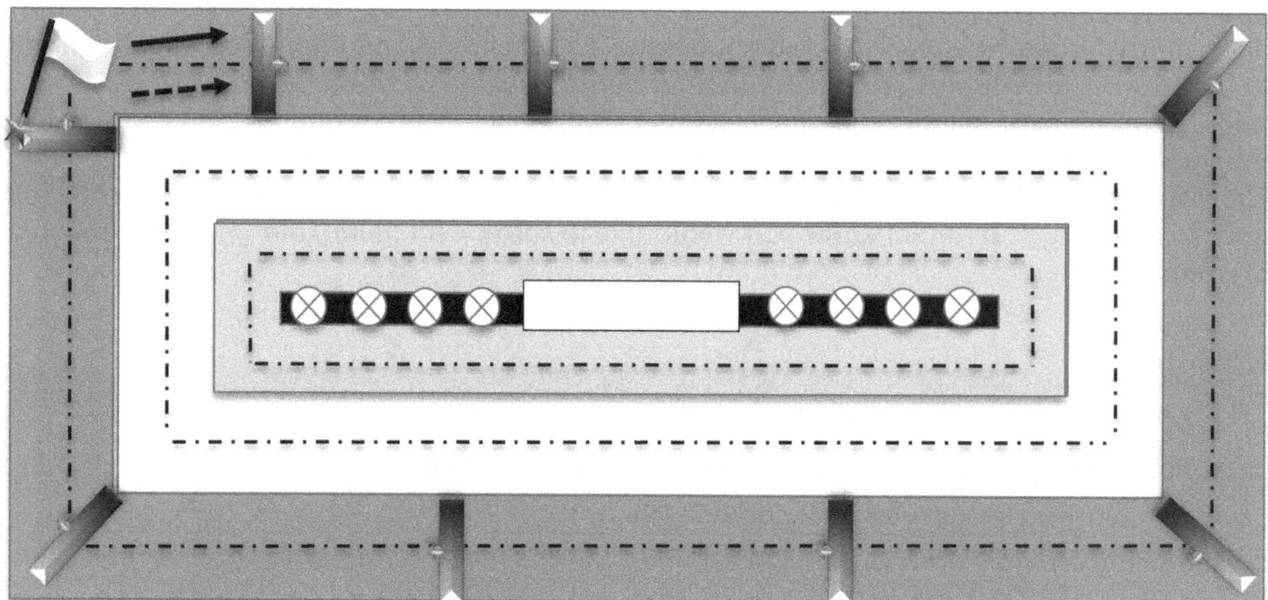

FIGURE 2–11. Staying on topic track.

- Choose a pen, pencil, or marker. Use different colors for each person, and draw any symbol (happy face, star, heart, or a solid arrow or a dashed-line arrow as shown) to make moves around the track.
- Each turn moves to the next stop post around the track.
- The winner is the person who goes around the outermost track and reaches the flag first or the person who stays out of the center if both players go off track.

- Each person decides if the conversational speaker (a) stayed on track (on topic) or spoke about a related topic or (b) went off topic (talking about something unrelated to what was said in the previous sentence).
- Introduce the topic. Any topic of interest is fine. For example, if in a room where there is a window, it is acceptable to start a conversation about the weather or what is going on outside or something to do outside.
- The first speaker can (a) share a photo readily available (from cell phone to start a topic of discussion), (b) look around the room and say something about something they see, or (c) choose from the conversation topics in Table 2–12.

A brief conversation:

Olivia: *I like the weather today. It's finally sunny outside. I would like to be outside.*

Ms. Jones: *Me too. I like when it's sunny too.* (On topic)

Olivia: *When I go home today, I'm going to take a walk outside.* (On topic)

Ms. Jones: *When I go home I have to cook dinner. What do you plan to do for dinner?*

(Related topic)

Olivia: *I'm not sure about dinner. We usually have pizza on Fridays. What about your dinner?* (On topic)

Ms. Jones: *I want to go to the movies.* (Off topic)

Ms. Jones: *Oh sorry, I should have told you about my dinner plans. I'm just so excited about the movies that I may forget to eat!* (Related topic)

Olivia: *That's OK. I do that all the time.* (On topic)

To Review

- Using the easy-hard chart (Figure 2–12), ask the child or teen, *"On a scale of 1 to 10 with 1 being very easy and 10 being very hard, how easy or hard was it to have the conversation? Choose a number from 1 to 10 to answer questions about the activity."*

TABLE 2–12. Possible Conversation Topics

■ What you want as a gift
■ Foods you like to eat and where you like to eat out
■ A game you like to play and how to play it
■ A show you like to watch and what it is about
■ A story about something that happened to you or a friend or your family

1 2 3 4 5 6 7 8 9 10

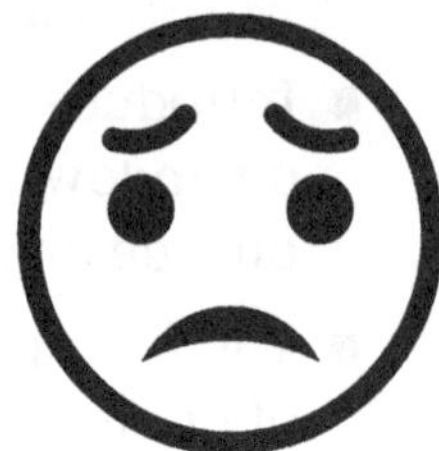

FIGURE 2–12. Easy-hard chart.

- *How easy or hard was it to stay focused on what I was saying?*
- *How easy or hard was it to think about what you were going to say?*
- *How easy or hard was it to stay relaxed?*
- *How easy or hard was it to decide if you should say the first thing you thought of?*
- *What did you like about the activity?*
- *What didn't you like about the activity?*

Suggestions to enhance treatment for children/teens with selective mutism can be found in Appendix 2–A, and suggestions to enhance treatment for stuttering can be found in Appendix 2–B, both at the end of Module 2.

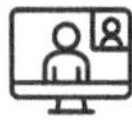
The online version of this activity includes an interactive game.

Activity Game 9: Conversation Wheelhouse

Goals of the Activity

- To attend to stories read aloud with pictures
- To share information and interact using the following eight conversational skills: (1) retelling, (2) questioning, (3) answering, (4) commenting, (5) sharing information, (6) telling a story/relating an event, (7) agreeing, and (8) disagreeing

In this activity, the child or teen works on conversational skills for story retelling, questioning, answering, commenting, sharing information, telling a story/relating an event, agreeing, and disagreeing. These skills are regularly incorporated into conversations and are spontaneous. Usually, the speaker does not know ahead of time the exact words they will say. Interchanges depend on what the conversational partners said previously.

Telling a story generally requires greater syntactic complexity (more advanced sentences) than when having a conversation (Nippold et al., 2014). What is easier about story narratives is that they usually follow a format and include a monologue that can be learned. Practice, rehearsal, and observation are beneficial. The following link provides videos of people engaged in conversational skills and can be used as demonstrations, where applicable. Open the link https://routledgetextbooks.com/textbooks/9781138238718/videos.php (Laugeson, 2017) to watch and discuss. Some video clips have both good and poor examples and can be used to identify what the actors could have done differently.

Materials

- Eight conversational skills with written explanations
- Situations to read with photos for role-plays (Figures 2–13 through 2–18)
- Conversational Skills Word Cards (Table 2–13)

Conversational Skills

1. Retelling—actively listening and attending to what others say so that you can retell the information.
    - Retell parts of a story you heard, something you read, or a program you watched.
2. Questioning—asking about something you want to know. Asking a question lets people know you are interested in what they say and that you want to know more.
    - Yes-No questions (i.e., Do/Does/Did, Am/Is/Are, Was/Were, Has/Have, Can/Could, Should, Would)
    - *Wh-* questions (i.e., Who, What, Where, When, Why, or How)
3. Answering—responding to someone who asked you a question. Answering lets people know you heard them and have something to share.
4. Commenting—saying a word, phrase, or sentence to let the speaker know you are listening and have some thoughts to share.
    - Comments help someone know what you think.
    - Comments help keep a conversation going.
    - Comments can add to a conversation by giving your *opinion,* saying how you *feel, agreeing* or *disagreeing,* sharing *information,* or giving *instructions,* stating an *intent* or *reason* for something, providing *clarification,* making a *prediction,* or offering a *suggestion,* to name several.
5. Sharing Information—providing information about anything that you would like to share.
    - This can include what you think, what you have done, or what you would like to do.
    - It can help someone learn how to do something new.
    - Sharing your thoughts and experiences usually helps someone else feel more comfortable.

6. Storytelling/relating events—telling a brief story or sharing an event about something that happened lets people know about your experiences. Stories have a beginning, middle, and end. When telling a story, try to include the following:
   - the people or characters (whom you are talking about)
   - the places or setting (where it took place)
   - what happened (the situation or events)
   - how the characters/people felt
   - if there was a problem or an issue
   - what was done to try to solve a problem
   - how things ended
7. Agreeing—letting someone know that you feel the same way as them and what they did or said.
   - People who agree with each other usually see things the same way.
8. Disagreeing—letting someone know that you see things differently than they do.
   - Letting someone know you have another way of looking at a situation or experience.

TABLE 2–13. Conversational Skills Word Cards

Retelling	Retelling	Pick-a-Card	Pick-a-Card
Questioning	Questioning	Pick-a-Card	Pick-a-Card
Answering	Answering	Pick-a-Card	Pick-a-Card
Commenting	Commenting	Pick-a-Card	Pick-a-Card
Sharing Information	Sharing Information	Pick-a-Card	Pick-a-Card
Storytelling Relating Events	Storytelling Relating Events	Pick-a-Card	Pick-a-Card
Agreeing	Agreeing	Pick-a-Card	Pick-a-Card
Disagreeing	Disagreeing	Pick-a-Card	Pick-a-Card

Situations With Photos

READ—The Situation: John

"This child, John, lives in my neighborhood. He's always getting in some type of trouble. I'm not sure if his parents pay attention to him because he runs around the neighborhood by himself. Maybe they think it's OK. I think he needs something to keep him busy and out of trouble."

1. Retelling—*Retell the information or the story you heard.*
2. Questioning—*Ask me a question related to the situation.*
3. Answering—*What do you think about this?*
4. Commenting—*Reply with a comment about what you think.*
5. Sharing Information—*Share something about yourself that is related to this situation.*
6. Storytelling/Relating Events—*Tell a brief story or relate an event about a similar situation.*
7. Agreeing—*Agree with something about the situation.*
8. Disagreeing—*Disagree with something about the situation.*

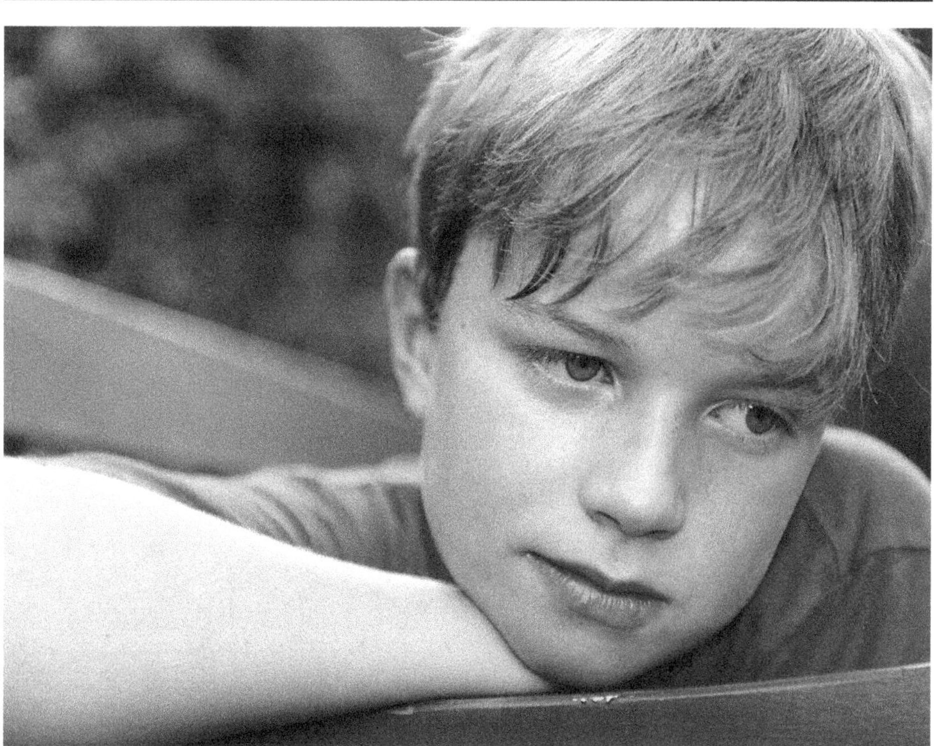

FIGURE 2–13. Situation role-play: John.

READ—The Situation: Play Ball

"The kids are at a playground having a great time. They are running to catch a ball. The boy in the black shirt is fast and it looks like he will catch that ball. If they are really playing soccer, there's a problem because no one is supposed to use their hands in a soccer game!"

1. Retelling—*Retell the information or the story you heard.*
2. Questioning—*Ask me a question related to the situation.*
3. Answering—*What do you think about this?*
4. Commenting—*Reply with a comment about what you think.*
5. Sharing Information—*Share something about yourself that is related to this situation.*
6. Storytelling/Relating Events—*Tell a brief story or relate an event about a similar situation.*
7. Agreeing—*Agree with something about the situation.*
8. Disagreeing—*Disagree with something about the situation.*

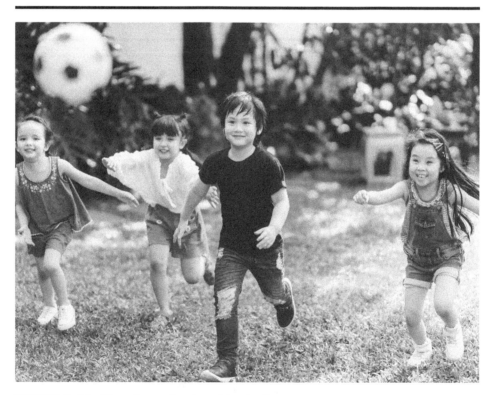

FIGURE 2–14. Situation role-play: Play ball.

READ—The Situation: Phone Girls

"These girls are good friends. Their names are Samantha and Joanne. They wanted to take a picture together, but no one was there to take it so they took a selfie. They must think they look good wearing their hats backward!"

1. Retelling—*Retell the information or the story you heard.*
2. Questioning—*Ask me a question related to the situation.*
3. Answering—*What do you think about this?*
4. Commenting—*Reply with a comment about what you think.*
5. Sharing Information—*Share something about yourself that is related to this situation.*
6. Storytelling/Relating Events—*Tell a brief story or relate an event about a similar situation.*
7. Agreeing—*Agree with something about the situation.*
8. Disagreeing—*Disagree with something about the situation.*

FIGURE 2–15. Situation role-play: Phone girls.

READ—The Situation: Workshop

"These seven students are planning a big event. They are planning a workshop about voting. All of them like political science and history. They are excited to plan the workshop for their school, and they are going to invite all students and families to join the online event to learn about voting."

1. Retelling—*Retell the information or the story you heard.*
2. Questioning—*Ask me a question related to the situation.*
3. Answering—*What do you think about this?*
4. Commenting—*Reply with a comment about what you think.*
5. Sharing Information—*Share something about yourself that is related to this situation.*
6. Storytelling/Relating Events—*Tell a brief story or relate an event about a similar situation.*
7. Agreeing—*Agree with something about the situation.*
8. Disagreeing—*Disagree with something about the situation.*

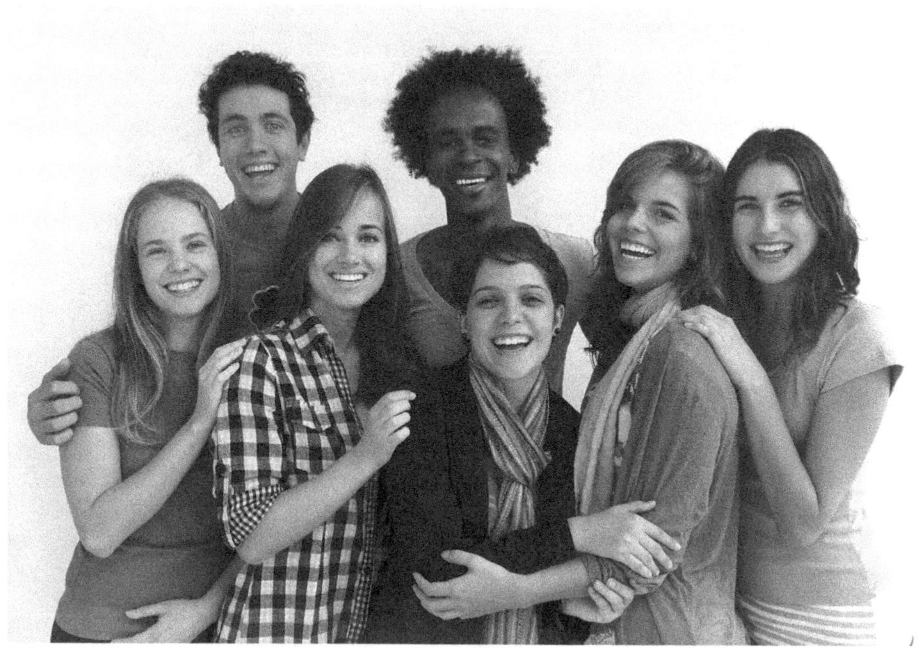

FIGURE 2–16. Situation role-play: Workshop.

READ—The Situation: Money

"The other day I found a brown paper bag on the sidewalk. I picked it up to throw it away, and it was filled with money. No one was around, and I didn't know what to do or how to find the real owner. I didn't feel right keeping the money because it wasn't mine."

1. Retelling—*Retell the information or the story you heard.*
2. Questioning—*Ask me a question related to the situation.*
3. Answering—*What do you think about this?*
4. Commenting—*Reply with a comment about what you think.*
5. Sharing Information—*Share something about yourself that is related to this situation.*
6. Storytelling/Relating Events—*Tell a brief story or relate an event about a similar situation.*
7. Agreeing—*Agree with something about the situation.*
8. Disagreeing—*Disagree with something about the situation.*

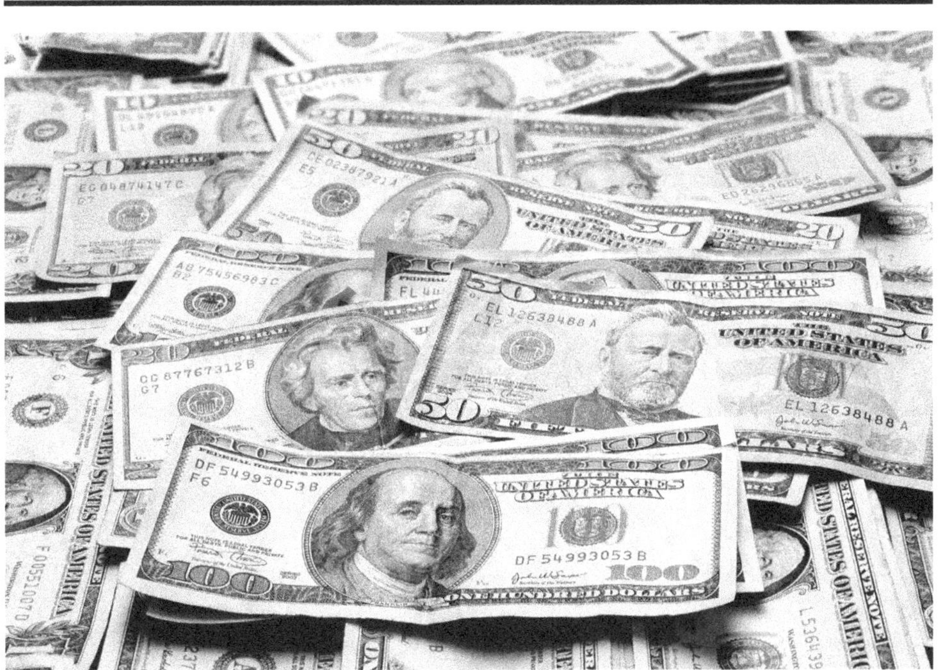

FIGURE 2–17. Situation role-play: Money.

READ—The Situation: Dinner

"This family is having a special holiday dinner together. There are parents and two kids, and they invited a friend and her daughter. They like to talk about their day. Everyone seems to like the food and they are having a good time."

1. Retelling—*Retell the information or the story you heard.*
2. Questioning—*Ask me a question related to the situation.*
3. Answering—*What do you think about this?*
4. Commenting—*Reply with a comment about what you think.*
5. Sharing Information—*Share something about yourself that is related to this situation.*
6. Storytelling/Relating Events—*Tell a brief story or relate an event about a similar situation.*
7. Agreeing—*Agree with something about the situation.*
8. Disagreeing—*Disagree with something about the situation.*

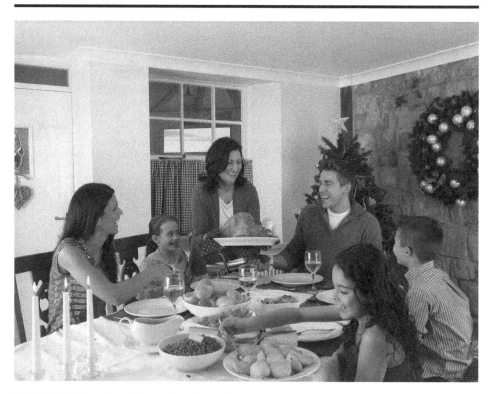

FIGURE 2–18. Situation role-play: Dinner.

How to Play

Cut the eight conversational skill words into separate cards and turn them face down (in Table 2–13). Cut the "Pick-a-Card" words into separate cards and place them on top of the conversational skill words so the words cannot be seen through the paper. You can also use tape or paste/glue to put the two blank sides together. Take turns picking a card and following the conversational skill after reading "The Situation." Choose as many scenes as you have time to practice, and engage in as many of the eight conversational skills as possible.

After all the scenes are completed, look around the current environment or place. What things do you see? Find an object you like or think about some topic to discuss. Ask the communication partner a question about it or make a comment about it to start a conversation.

Keep track of how many conversational skills were used.

_____ Retelling information or story	_____ Sharing information
_____ Asking a question	_____ Telling a story/relating events
_____ Answering a question	_____ Agreeing
_____ Making a comment	_____ Disagreeing

If any of the tasks pose difficulty, the facilitator can model an example or provide a response for the child or teen and then reenact the task for practice.

Suggestions to enhance treatment for children/teens with selective mutism can be found in Appendix 2–A, and suggestions to enhance treatment for stuttering can be found in Appendix 2–B, both at the end of Module 2.

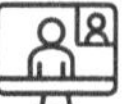

The online version of this activity includes an interactive game.

Activity Game 10: Conversational Role-Plays: Pragmatic Language

Goals of the Activity

The following 10 pragmatic language skills are frequently found in daily conversations and interactions. The goals in this activity are to increase use of the following:

1. Greetings/hello/opening a conversation—saying *Hi; How are you?; What's new; Do you have a minute?; Can we talk?;* etc.
2. Leaving/goodbyes/closing a conversation—saying *Bye; See you later; I have to go now; I won't keep you; Good talking to you;* etc.
3. Thanking/showing appreciation—saying *Thanks; Thank you for . . . ; I appreciate what you said; I appreciate what you did;* etc.
4. Commenting or complimenting—commenting on what someone else did or said: *I like your . . . ; That was really nice; You helped me . . . ; That's good; That's interesting;* etc.
5. Apologizing—saying *I'm sorry, I apologize, I didn't mean to . . . ;* for doing or saying something you wish you didn't do or say, etc.
6. Requesting clarification or information—asking a question such as: *Can you explain . . . ; Can you tell me . . . ; Can you let me know more about . . . ; What . . . ;* etc., to gather information you need or want.
7. Stating a problem or making an excuse—letting someone know there is a problem by expressing your needs or point of view: *There seems to be a problem with . . . ; I need to talk to you about something; I'm sorry something isn't working out;* or *I didn't mean for this to happen . . . ;* etc.
8. Making a complaint or complaining—saying what bothers you or what has been done wrong: *I want you to know something; I'm going to need your help; Something has to be changed; I need to tell you about . . . ; We have a problem with . . . ;* etc.
9. Asking for help or offering help—saying: *Can you help me . . . ; I need to ask if you can help me with . . . ; If it isn't too much trouble, can you . . . ;* or *Is there something I can help you with; I might be able to help you with that;* etc.
10. Providing information—giving someone information about an experience, event, or sharing knowledge about a topic: *Let me tell you about . . . ; Something interesting happened to me that I'd like to tell you;* or giving someone information or instruction such as: *I can tell you how . . . ; I have something to tell you.*

In this activity, the child or teen works on specific pragmatic language skills for opening and closing a conversation, showing appreciation, commenting, complimenting, apologizing, requesting clarification/information, stating a problem, making an excuse, making a complaint, asking for help or offering help, and providing information. These speech acts are often used in everyday interactions.

As these social pragmatic skills are practiced, let the child/teen know that they may feel a little anxious when engaging in some new interactions but that it is necessary to gain experience and reduce avoidance. If they feel nervous, remind them that those feelings are natural and normal. Encourage them to greet their anxiety by saying to themselves, *"This is me feeling a little nervous. I am about to do something that I haven't done much before, but I can do it!"* Suggest they take an easy breath in and let it out slowly, quietly, and calmly. Add the thought, *"I am going to say something, and there is no right or wrong way. It just is."* The less pressure the child or teen puts on themself, the better they will feel, and the more chances they will take to participate in spontaneous conversations. Reinforce the idea of focusing on the present moment and what they want to do or say instead of possibly worrying about it.

A social monitoring form may be useful to help the child or teen better understand what places, situations, or people make them feel uneasy or less likely to communicate. How the child or teen feels, what they think, and what they do about communicating can help them gain insight into the patterns that influence their behaviors. In each situation, complete the sentence:

If I was ________ (identify situation and role) ________, I would probably feel (feeling word) ________, because I think ________ (what may happen) ________, and then I would ________ (what end up doing) ________.

If the child/teen cannot fill in the blanks for the situation, give choices that are common possibilities. For example, using Topic 15 in the scenes that follow (student at school needs help with the computer), the child/teen may generate the following sentence completion with your assistance:

If I was at school and my computer wasn't working, I would probably feel nervous about asking the teacher for help, because I think the teacher might think I broke it, and then I would get in trouble.

Given the output from the child/teen, the facilitator may be able to problem-solve the situation and present alternatives.

Materials

- Topics and roles for 15 scenarios
- Photos—Figures 2–19 through 2–33
- Checklist of selected social language skills

Topics, Roles, and Photos for Scenarios

Topic 1—Providing information, making an excuse, apologizing, and commenting

Roles—(1) Homeowner who answers door, (2) Person who threw the ball and broke the window by mistake

Who do you want to be and what will you say?

Check off the social pragmatic language skills used in the role-play.

1. ____ Greetings, saying hello, opening a conversation (to do each conversation)
2. ____ Leaving, saying goodbyes, closing a conversation (to do each conversation)
3. ____ Thanking, showing appreciation
4. ____ Commenting, complimenting
5. ____ Apologizing
6. ____ Requesting clarification or information
7. ____ Stating a problem or making an excuse
8. ____ Making a complaint or complaining
9. ____ Asking for help or offering help
10. ____ Providing information

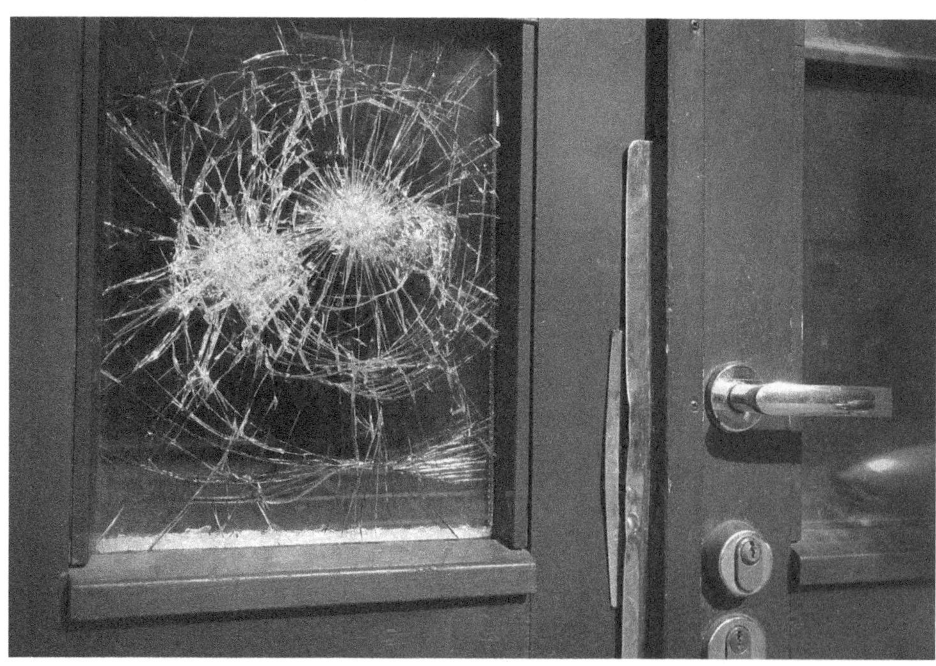

FIGURE 2–19. Breaking a window.

Topic 2—Commenting, stating a problem, apologizing, and thanking

Roles—(1) Cashier at the store taking money; (2) person paying for the item does not get the correct change from the cashier

Who do you want to be and what will you say?

Check off the social pragmatic language skills used in the role-play.

1. ____ Greetings, saying hello, opening a conversation (to do each conversation)
2. ____ Leaving, saying goodbyes, closing a conversation (to do each conversation)
3. ____ Thanking, showing appreciation
4. ____ Commenting, complimenting
5. ____ Apologizing
6. ____ Requesting clarification or information
7. ____ Stating a problem or making an excuse
8. ____ Making a complaint or complaining
9. ____ Asking for help or offering help
10. ____ Providing information

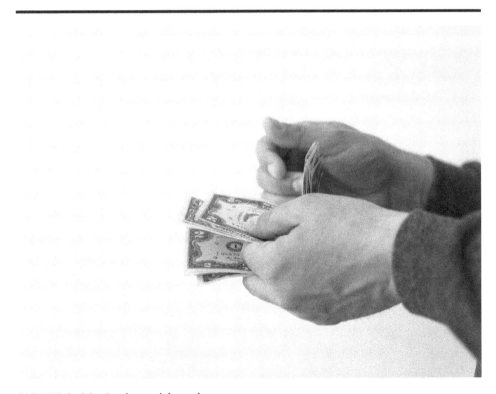

FIGURE 2–20. Paying with cash.

Topic 3—Providing information, stating a problem, asking for help, offering help, and thanking

Roles—(1) Teacher leading class is giving instructions, (2) student in the group cannot do the exercises because of feeling sick

Who do you want to be, and what will you say?

Check off the social pragmatic language skills used in the role-play.

1. ____ Greetings, saying hello, opening a conversation (to do each conversation)
2. ____ Leaving, saying goodbyes, closing a conversation (to do each conversation)
3. ____ Thanking, showing appreciation
4. ____ Commenting, complimenting
5. ____ Apologizing
6. ____ Requesting clarification or information
7. ____ Stating a problem or making an excuse
8. ____ Making a complaint or complaining
9. ____ Asking for help or offering help
10. ____ Providing information

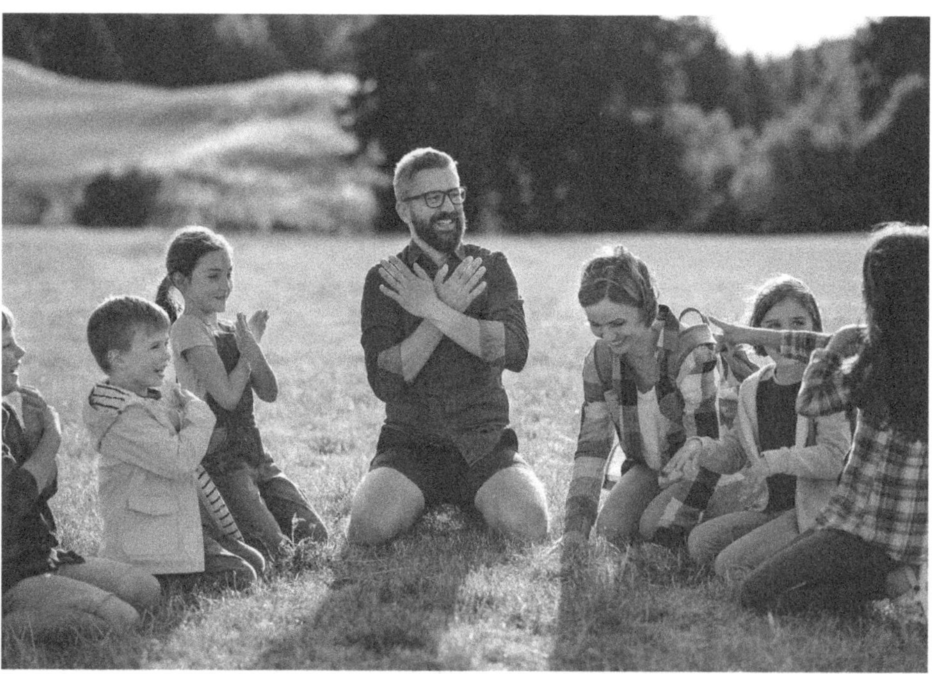

FIGURE 2–21. Teacher leading the class.

Topic 4—Requesting clarification, providing information, and showing appreciation

Roles—(1) Younger girl pulling the gift toward herself, (2) older girl saying the gift is hers

Who do you want to be, and what will you say?

Check off the social pragmatic language skills used in the role-play.

1. ____ Greetings, saying hello, opening a conversation (to do each conversation)
2. ____ Leaving, saying goodbyes, closing a conversation (to do each conversation)
3. ____ Thanking, showing appreciation
4. ____ Commenting, complimenting
5. ____ Apologizing
6. ____ Requesting clarification or information
7. ____ Stating a problem or making an excuse
8. ____ Making a complaint or complaining
9. ____ Asking for help or offering help
10. ____ Providing information

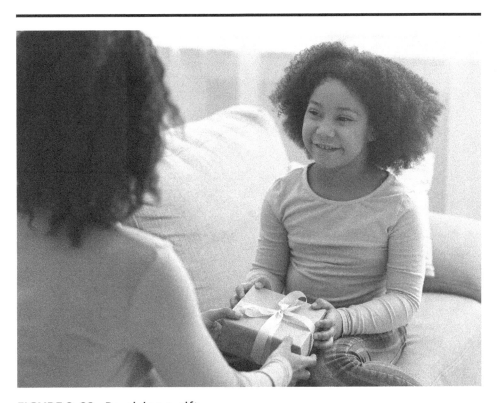

FIGURE 2–22. Receiving a gift.

Topic 5—Stating a problem, providing information, and offering help

Roles—(1) Driver of the car is heading down the wrong street, (2) passenger in the car lets the driver know she is going the wrong way and how she should go to her friend's house

Who do you want to be and what will you say?

Check off the social pragmatic language skills used in the role-play.

1. ____ Greetings, saying hello, opening a conversation (to do each conversation)
2. ____ Leaving, saying goodbyes, closing a conversation (to do each conversation)
3. ____ Thanking, showing appreciation
4. ____ Commenting, complimenting
5. ____ Apologizing
6. ____ Requesting clarification or information
7. ____ Stating a problem or making an excuse
8. ____ Making a complaint or complaining
9. ____ Asking for help or offering help
10. ____ Providing information

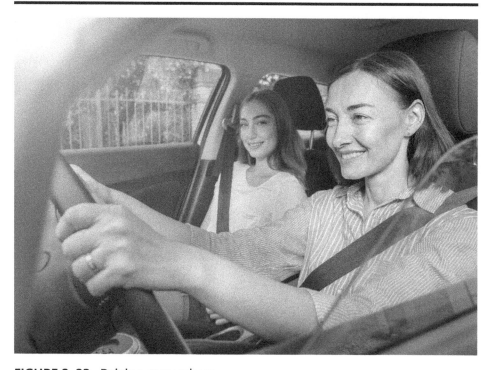

FIGURE 2–23. Driving somewhere.

Topic 6—Asking for help, making a complaint, commenting, and thanking

Roles—(1) Adult is trying to help the child with his homework, (2) child doesn't think the adult is doing the homework correctly

Who do you want to be and what will you say?

Check off the social pragmatic language skills used in the role-play.

1. ____ Greetings, saying hello, opening a conversation (to do each conversation)
2. ____ Leaving, saying goodbyes, closing a conversation (to do each conversation)
3. ____ Thanking, showing appreciation
4. ____ Commenting, complimenting
5. ____ Apologizing
6. ____ Requesting clarification or information
7. ____ Stating a problem or making an excuse
8. ____ Making a complaint or complaining
9. ____ Asking for help or offering help
10. ____ Providing information

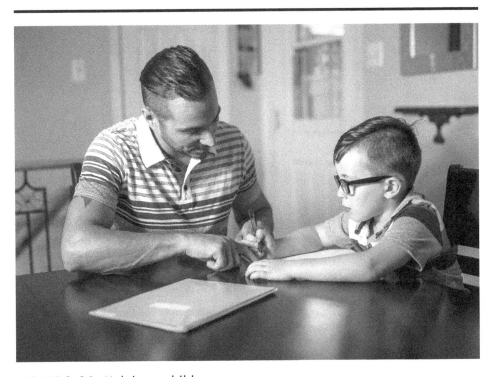

FIGURE 2–24. Helping a child.

Topic 7—Providing information, commenting, and showing appreciation

Roles—(1) Grandmother lets child know she likes flowers but not in her hair, (2) the child tells her grandmother what she thinks about flowers

Who do you want to be and what will you say?

Check off the social pragmatic language skills used in the role-play.

1. ____ Greetings, saying hello, opening a conversation (to do each conversation)
2. ____ Leaving, saying goodbyes, closing a conversation (to do each conversation)
3. ____ Thanking, showing appreciation
4. ____ Commenting, complimenting
5. ____ Apologizing
6. ____ Requesting clarification or information
7. ____ Stating a problem or making an excuse
8. ____ Making a complaint or complaining
9. ____ Asking for help or offering help
10. ____ Providing information

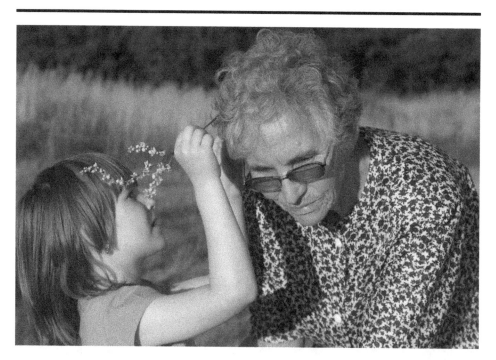

FIGURE 2–25. Picking flowers.

Topic 8—Providing information, making an excuse, and commenting

Roles—(1) Child tells his family that he found their dog who ran away, (2) parent talks to child about taking care of the dog

Who do you want to be, and what will you say?

Check off the social pragmatic language skills used in the role-play.

1. ____ Greetings, saying hello, opening a conversation (to do each conversation)
2. ____ Leaving, saying goodbyes, closing a conversation (to do each conversation)
3. ____ Thanking, showing appreciation
4. ____ Commenting, complimenting
5. ____ Apologizing
6. ____ Requesting clarification or information
7. ____ Stating a problem or making an excuse
8. ____ Making a complaint or complaining
9. ____ Asking for help or offering help
10. ____ Providing information

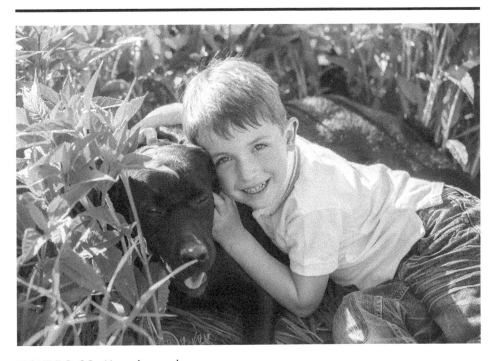

FIGURE 2–26. Hugging a dog.

Topic 9—Requesting information, providing information, and commenting

Roles—(1) Teacher asks students where they want to go for an upcoming class trip, (2) students answer the teacher

Who do you want to be and what will you say?

Check off the social pragmatic language skills used in the role-play.

1. ____ Greetings, saying hello, opening a conversation (to do each conversation)
2. ____ Leaving, saying goodbyes, closing a conversation (to do each conversation)
3. ____ Thanking, showing appreciation
4. ____ Commenting, complimenting
5. ____ Apologizing
6. ____ Requesting clarification or information
7. ____ Stating a problem or making an excuse
8. ____ Making a complaint or complaining
9. ____ Asking for help or offering help
10. ____ Providing information

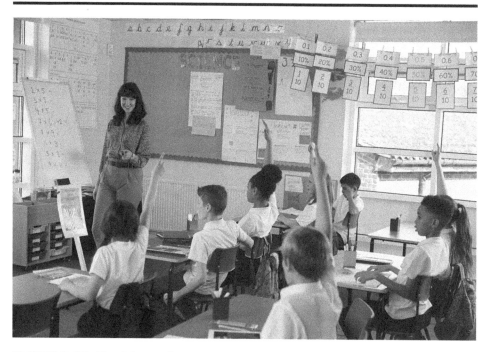

FIGURE 2–27. Teaching a class.

Topic 10—Stating a problem, making a complaint, and commenting

Roles—(1) Nurse is telling a mother that her child cannot go to school for at least another week, (2) child tells mother she is worried about missing school for so many days

Who do you want to be, and what will you say?

Check off the social pragmatic language skills used in the role-play.

1. ____ Greetings, saying hello, opening a conversation (to do each conversation)
2. ____ Leaving, saying goodbyes, closing a conversation (to do each conversation)
3. ____ Thanking, showing appreciation
4. ____ Commenting, complimenting
5. ____ Apologizing
6. ____ Requesting clarification or information
7. ____ Stating a problem or making an excuse
8. ____ Making a complaint or complaining
9. ____ Asking for help or offering help
10. ____ Providing information

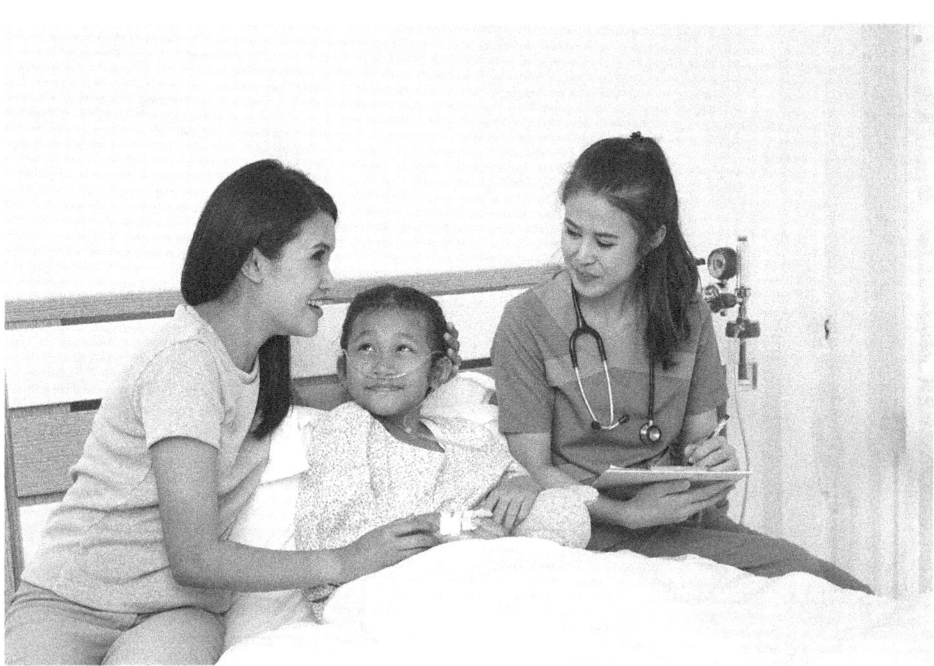

FIGURE 2–28. Helping a sick child.

Topic 11— Stating a problem, complaining, and apologizing

Roles—(1) Dog walker has to tell the owner one of the dogs ran away, (2) owner is going to be very upset

Who do you want to be, and what will you say?

Check off the social pragmatic language skills used in the role-play.

1. ____ Greetings, saying hello, opening a conversation (to do each conversation)
2. ____ Leaving, saying goodbyes, closing a conversation (to do each conversation)
3. ____ Thanking, showing appreciation
4. ____ Commenting, complimenting
5. ____ Apologizing
6. ____ Requesting clarification or information
7. ____ Stating a problem or making an excuse
8. ____ Making a complaint or complaining
9. ____ Asking for help or offering help
10. ____ Providing information

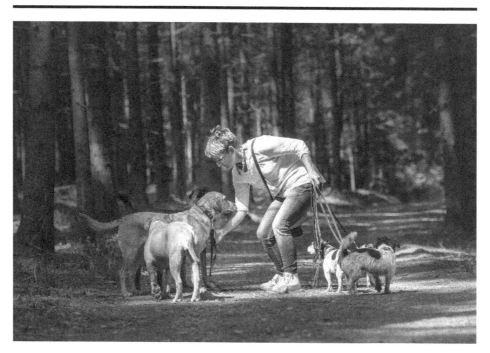

FIGURE 2–29. Walking dogs.

Topic 12—Making a complaint, apologizing, offering help, and showing appreciation

Roles—(1) Someone in family tells server they didn't order coffee, (2) server apologizes and asks what she can bring

Who do you want to be, and what will you say?

Check off the social pragmatic language skills used in the role-play.

1. ____ Greetings, saying hello, opening a conversation (to do each conversation)
2. ____ Leaving, saying goodbyes, closing a conversation (to do each conversation)
3. ____ Thanking, showing appreciation
4. ____ Commenting, complimenting
5. ____ Apologizing
6. ____ Requesting clarification or information
7. ____ Stating a problem or making an excuse
8. ____ Making a complaint or complaining
9. ____ Asking for help or offering help
10. ____ Providing information

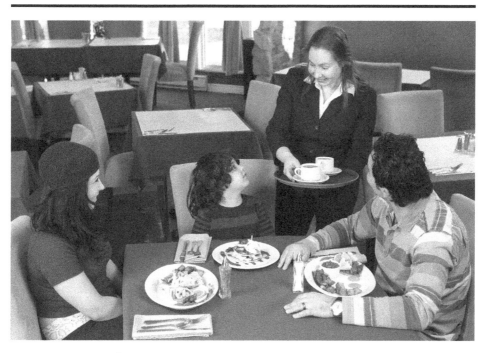

FIGURE 2–30. Ordering in restaurant.

Topic 13—Providing information, making a complaint, apologizing, and commenting

Roles—(1) Customers tell server what they want to order, (2) server behind counter gives them the wrong food

Who do you want to be, and what will you say?

Check off the social pragmatic language skills used in the role-play.

1. ____ Greetings, saying hello, opening a conversation (to do each conversation)
2. ____ Leaving, saying goodbyes, closing a conversation (to do each conversation)
3. ____ Thanking, showing appreciation
4. ____ Commenting, complimenting
5. ____ Apologizing
6. ____ Requesting clarification or information
7. ____ Stating a problem or making an excuse
8. ____ Making a complaint or complaining
9. ____ Asking for help or offering help
10. ____ Providing information

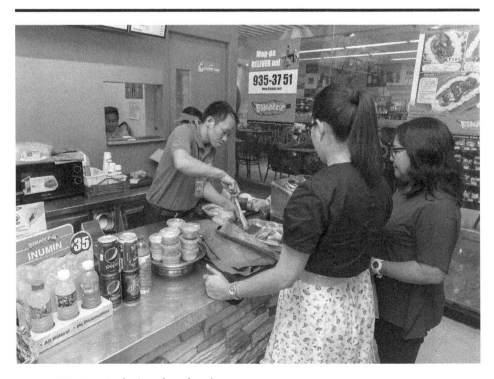

FIGURE 2–31. Ordering fast food.

Topic 14—Commenting, asking for help, offering help, and showing appreciation

Roles—(1) Person buying the food doesn't have enough money to pay, (2) cashier is trying to help her get the right amount of food so that she can pay for everything

Who do you want to be, and what will you say?

Check off the social pragmatic language skills used in the role-play.

1. ____ Greetings, saying hello, opening a conversation (to do each conversation)
2. ____ Leaving, saying goodbyes, closing a conversation (to do each conversation)
3. ____ Thanking, showing appreciation
4. ____ Commenting, complimenting
5. ____ Apologizing
6. ____ Requesting clarification or information
7. ____ Stating a problem or making an excuse
8. ____ Making a complaint or complaining
9. ____ Asking for help or offering help
10. ____ Providing information

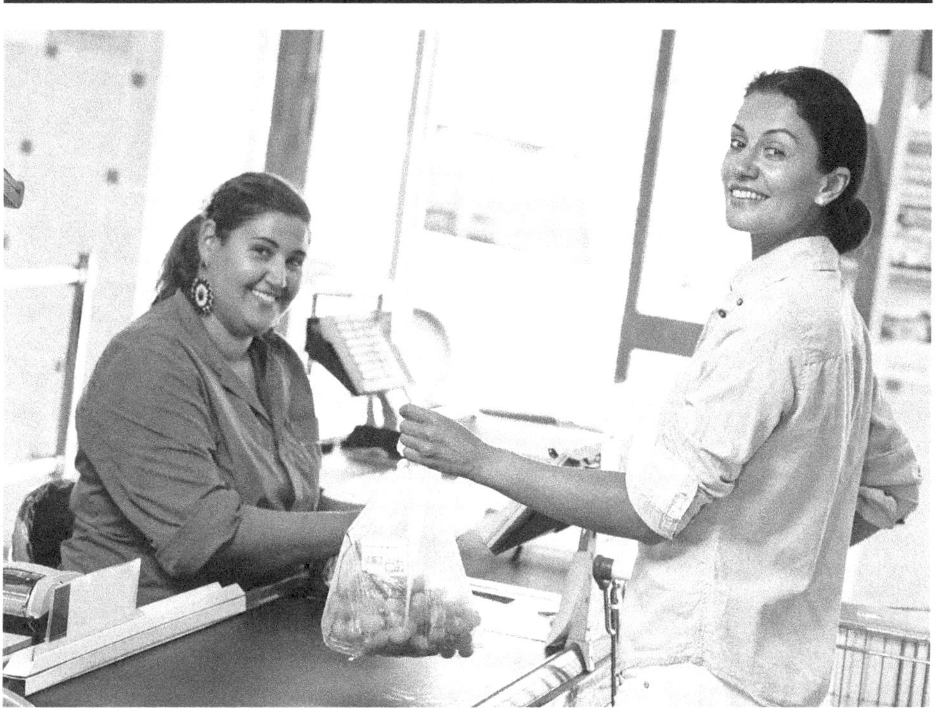

FIGURE 2–32. Buying food.

Topic 15—Stating a problem, commenting, offering help, and showing appreciation

Roles—(1) Student tells teaching assistant that the computer is broken and that she can't finish her work, (2) teaching assistant tries to help her

Who do you want to be, and what will you say?

Check off the social pragmatic language skills used in the role-play.

1. ____ Greetings, saying hello, opening a conversation (to do each conversation)
2. ____ Leaving, saying goodbyes, closing a conversation (to do each conversation)
3. ____ Thanking, showing appreciation
4. ____ Commenting, complimenting
5. ____ Apologizing
6. ____ Requesting clarification or information
7. ____ Stating a problem or making an excuse
8. ____ Making a complaint or complaining
9. ____ Asking for help or offering help
10. ____ Providing information

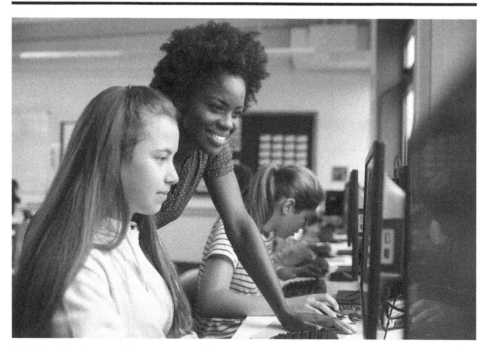

FIGURE 2–33. Getting computer help.

How to Play

Introduce the 10 social pragmatic language skills for the role-plays. Provide some examples from daily encounters. Keep the page with the skills in view for the child/teen to recall. It may be that the child/teen only uses a few of the 10 skills in daily encounters and in the role-plays provided. To increase their repertoire, provide an example as appropriate to the role-play and ask the child or teen to imitate the facilitator (for their turn). Work toward using all 10 skills, if appropriate to the specific role-play scene. Each time a speaker engages in one of the 10 skills, put a check mark next to that skill on the list to track progress. To engage in this activity do the following:

1. Look at the photo and analyze what has happened and what may happen next. Talk about it briefly. The facilitator is encouraged to use *think-alouds* as a strategy to actually say what they are thinking so that the child/teen can hear how the facilitator is processing the scenario and what they may do to try to accomplish the task or solve the issue. For example, in Topic 13 (scenario where the server behind the counter gives the people the wrong food), the facilitator can use the think-aloud process to say the following:

   The customer in the black shirt is thinking, wow, the server gave me the wrong meal. This isn't what I ordered. I'm not going to eat this. I shouldn't have to pay for this. I better say something to the man so he can give me the food I actually ordered. What if he doesn't give me the right food? I'm not going to eat this or pay for it if it's not my order. I have to tell him this is the wrong order for me and give him my order again. I hope he will fix it. Luckily my friend got what she ordered.
2. Before beginning each role-play, select several pragmatic language skills from the list that seem to fit the scene. Try all 10 if they apply.
3. Choose roles that each person wants to play or act out. Explain that this activity is like being an actor. Actors take on different roles and try to portray different people.
4. One person starts or initiates the scene. Decide on this ahead of time.
5. Each player should say what comes to their mind based on the situation.
6. If not sure what to say, use Table 2–14 to help organize those thoughts. The child/teen can also imitate what the facilitator says or suggests.
7. Reenact the scene again to get more comfortable after practicing. Take turns switching roles using the 15 topics, roles, and photos. Add pictures or share photos to create sample scenarios for the role-plays.

Relating Acting to Real-Life Encounters

After finishing all the topics and role-plays, try a situation that the child/teen would like to role-play, one that they may have encountered. List the topic and roles first. Ask if the child or teen has a photo they can share to give a visual of the scene. The Dreamstime website (https://www.dreamstime.com/) or other stock picture websites have a multitude of realistic photos to search.

TABLE 2–14. Questions to Help Organize Thoughts

What do I already know about this?	What questions could I ask?
What else do I want to know?	What can I share about this topic?

Act out scenes that are encountered in the child/teen's life. Real possibilities may include ordering ice cream or donuts from a neighborhood store, ordering from a take-out or drive-thru restaurant, or speaking to a salesperson at a store to get something, or asking someone at school to get permission to go to the bathroom, or get help with an assignment.

- Set the scene by asking the child/teen questions about the situation. First engage in a practice role-play. For example, if using an ice cream shop scene, you can ask the child/teen what they would like to order and what they would need to say when the person behind the counter asks them, "What kind of ice cream would you like?"
- Add details such as the ice cream shop has 25 flavors. Tell the child/teen to ask if they can sample one of the flavors. Act out that part, and have the child/teen choose a flavor, choose a type of cone, ask how much it costs, pay the person, and then say thank you. Try to make the role-play as realistic a scene as they may encounter. Check out the link, https://www.dreamstime.com/photos-images/ice-cream-shop.html
- During the next week or so, ask the child/teen to go with their parent or guardian to a store and buy ice cream, recalling the practice scene. The facilitator will need to speak with the adult (parent/guardian) to set this up ahead of time.
- Reduce the urge to engage in rescuing behaviors (speaking for the child/teen so they can get what they want). This negative reinforcement cycle perpetuates avoidance. Let the child know that they need to ask for the flavor they want in order to get their ice cream (or to acquire other things as the situations present themselves).
- Table 2–14 can help the child/teen think about a scene and organize their thoughts prior to enacting it.

Suggestions to enhance treatment for children/teens with selective mutism can be found in Appendix 2–A, and suggestions to enhance treatment for stuttering can be found in Appendix 2–B, both at the end of Module 2.

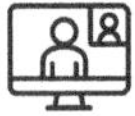

The online version of this activity includes an interactive game.

Activity Game 11: Chat Spin—Informal Conversations

Goals of the Activity

- To increase conversational skills to:
  1. Take turns listening and speaking
  2. Keep the conversation going by asking questions, giving answers, and making comments
  3. Share experiences, thoughts, and opinions
  4. Use expression in your voice
  5. Smile or act interested in what the other person says

This activity provides experiences for engaging in an informal chat about various topics. Chats are informal conversations based on familiar topics and mutual interests. They are usually composed of open dialogue without judgment. Fear of negative evaluation or worry about being judged can be a powerful force and limit one's attempts and ultimate willingness to engage in a chat or conversation. Perfectionistic tendences can create high achievement goals and can also lead to a lack of satisfaction and self-criticism. Sometimes unrealistic standards are set that can prevent people from attempting tasks because they cannot accept anything less than what they think is perfect. According to Amster and Klein (2018), *self-oriented perfectionists* are critical of themselves when their own expectations are thought to be unmet. *Other-oriented perfectionists* want perfection of themselves because they think that is what others expect of them, and if they don't reach those standards, they think others will judge them poorly. Making mistakes can be scary to someone with socially prescribed perfectionism (Melero et al., 2020). Mistakes are a natural part of learning and help people grow in many areas of functioning, including communication.

Materials

- Pre-Chat Review (Table 2–15)
- Role-playing topics for conversation (Table 2–16)
- Wheel 1: Topics for Conversation—Words (Figure 2–34)
- Wheel 2: Topics for Conversation—Sentences (Figure 2–35)
- Post-Chat Review (Table 2–17)

Play a guessing game. One person thinks of their response, and the other person tries to guess what they will say.

How to Play

Tell the child or teen that you are going to chat. A chat is an informal conversation. People say what comes to their mind. Chatting is like texting where you share information.

1. When people chat using spoken words, the words are fleeting. As soon as they are said they are gone, and people often do not remember the exact words that were said. They

remember the ideas. In texting, the words last and can be reviewed in print. That can give people more time to plan what to share. The child or teen may want to text at times if they have a smartphone. They can also practice by reading texts aloud.

2. Before starting, fill in the Pre-Chat Review.
3. Cut the conversation topics into squares (Table 2–16) or cut the paper sections from Wheel 1 (Figure 2–34). Fold the papers and mix them up. Pick a paper. The players can also close their eyes and without looking, point to a topic on the wheel. Start a chat about the chosen topic. Take turns.
4. Also play Wheel 2 (Figure 2–35) with sentences. Cut the sections and fold the papers, mixing them up. Select one. If there is someone who knows the child or teen well and can be part of the activity, include them. Ask that familiar person to take turns guessing answers that they think the child/teen would give. They should write their answer and check to see if they were correct after the other person gives their answer. Take turns guessing.

Suggestions to enhance treatment for children/teens with selective mutism can be found in Appendix 2–A, and suggestions to enhance treatment for stuttering can be found in Appendix 2–B, both at the end of Module 2.

The online version of this activity includes an interactive game.

TABLE 2–15. Pre-Chat Fill-in-the Blanks

1. When I share information with someone, I ______________________.
2. When someone asks me a question, I ______________________.
3. The topics I like to talk about are ______________________.
4. When someone else is talking, I ______________________.
5. When I am speaking with someone, I wonder ______________________.
6. When speaking with someone, I want to ______________________.
7. I notice that when I have something to say, people ______________________.
8. I ask other people questions when ______________________.
9. When chatting with someone, I want to get better at ______________________.
10. When chatting with someone, I think I am getting better at ______________________.

TABLE 2–16. 20 Topics for Conversations

Pets	Food
School	Music
Friends	Sports
Hobbies	Good time
Jobs	Travel
Dentist	TV show
Weather	Video game
Weekends	Vacation
Free time	Gifts
Homes	Birthday
Amusement rides	Wish
Topic of your choice	Topic of your choice

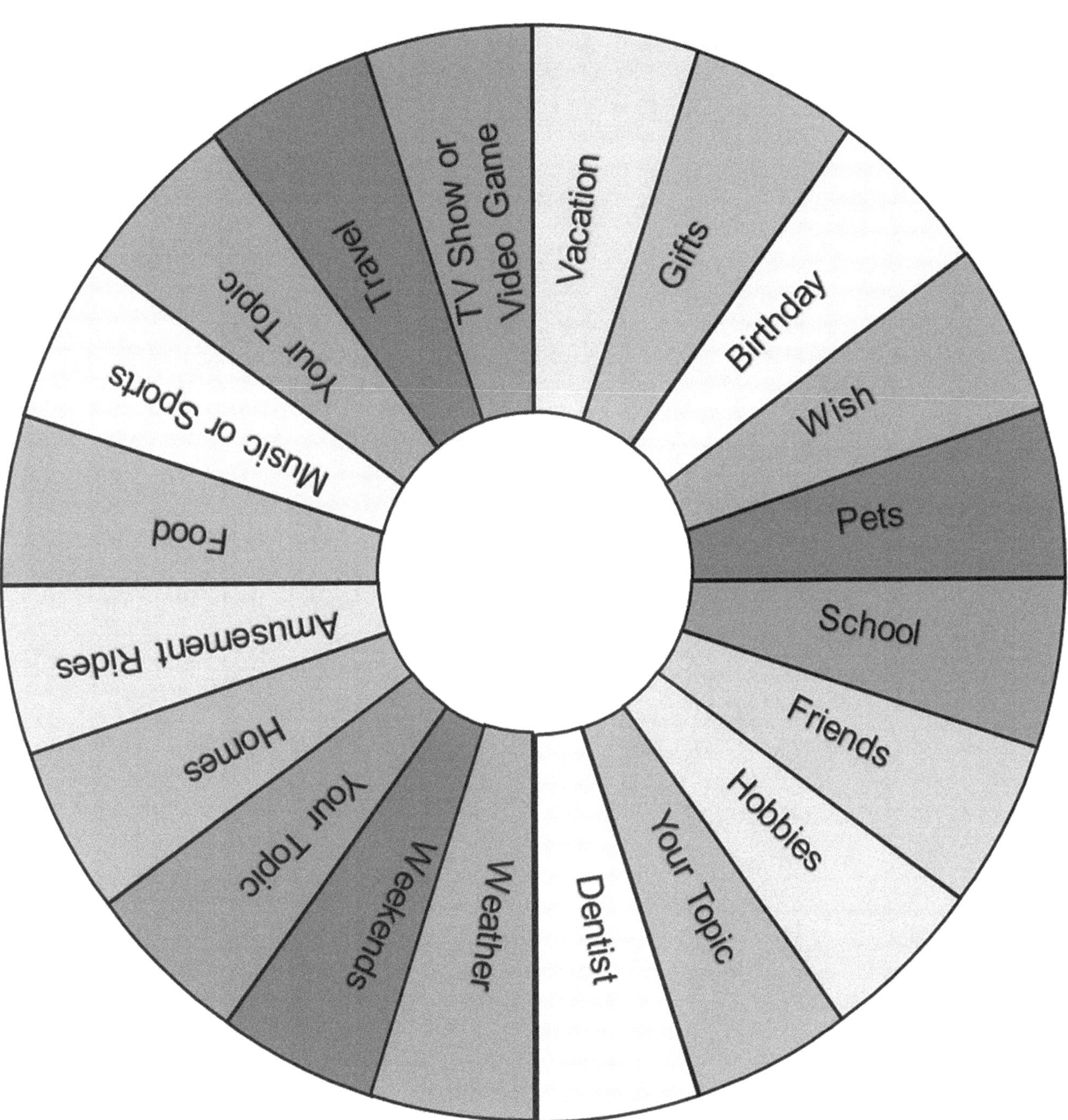

FIGURE 2–34. Wheel 1: Topics for Conversation—Words. Chat about a topic.

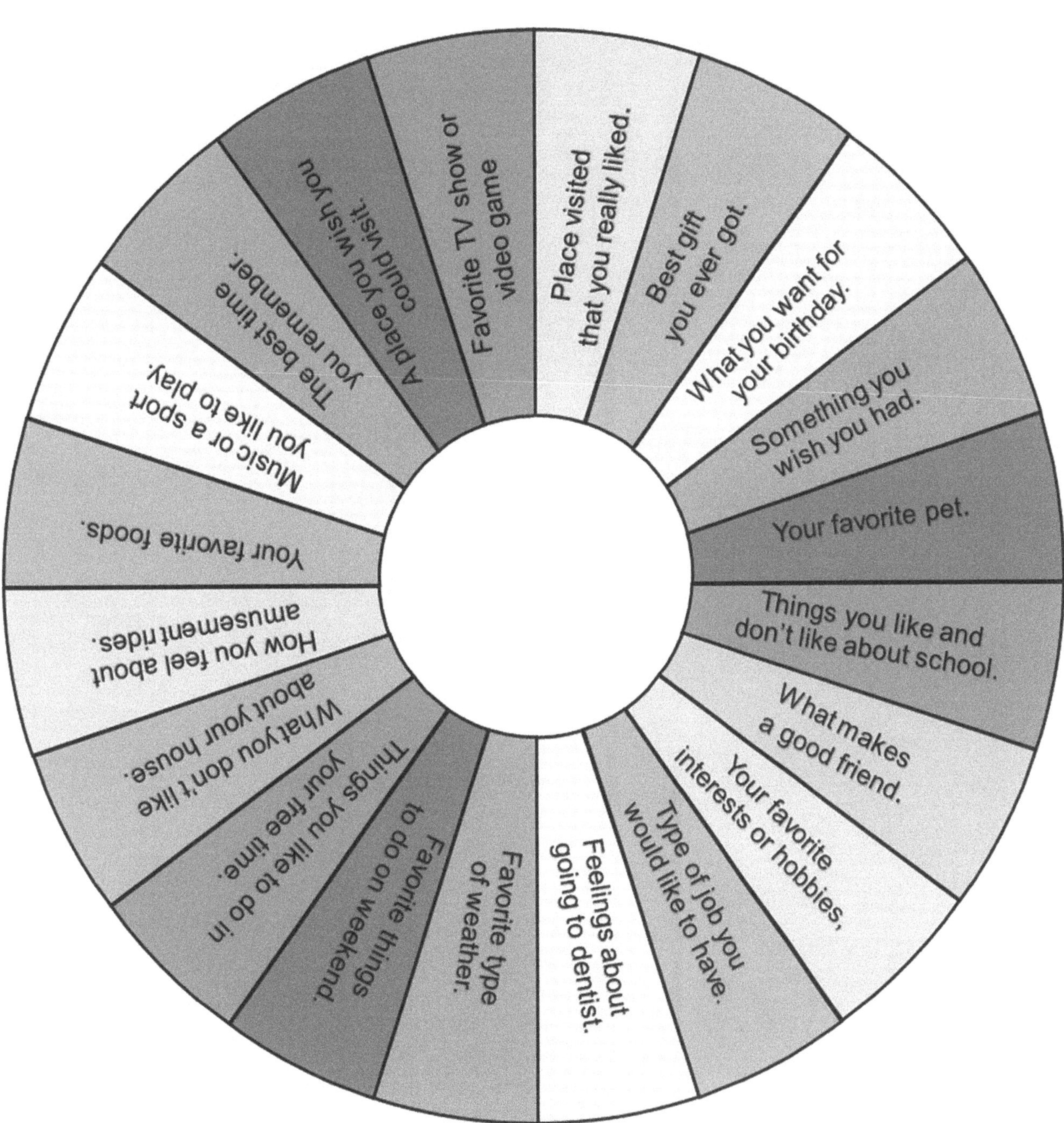

FIGURE 2–35. Wheel 2: Topics for Conversation—Sentences.

TABLE 2–17. Post-Chat Fill-in-the Blanks Review

1. When I shared information with you, I ________________.
2. When you asked me a question, I ________________.
3. The topics I liked to talk about were ________________.
4. When you spoke, I found myself ________________.
5. When I spoke with you, I wondered ________________.
6. When I spoke with you, I wanted to ________________.
7. I noticed that when I had something to say, you ________________.
8. I thought the topics were ________________.
9. When chatting with you, I wanted to get better at ________________.
10. When chatting with you, I thought I was getting better at ________________.

Module 2: Outreach Activities

The activities that follow were created for the facilitator and child/teen to gain experience working on personalized outreach skills. During this time, it can be helpful if the facilitator and/or significant others in the child or teen's life unobtrusively observe interactional skills during outreach activities. Doing so can help the facilitator work on needed social skills for interacting with peers and others in their environment. Programs by Elizabeth Laugeson, Michelle Garcia Winner, and Jed Baker, to name a few, include social skills work and can provide additional experiences.

The following sections can be implemented to increase personally functional communication within the individual's environment.

Ordering From Stores: Donut Shop, Ice Cream Shop, Restaurant, Store, Etc.

1. Secure a picture related to the place (storefront, menu, or items for sale from that specific place on the Internet or from a pamphlet).
2. Decide what the child/teen wants to find out and write the questions to ask and rehearse them.
3. Using the phone or in-person, ask your question.
4. The questions can include what time the place is open, if the place has a specific item or food to order.
5. Role-play the scene with the child or teen. Decide on the roles and then take turns. Switch so each person can speak as the shopkeeper or restaurant server and patron/shopper.
6. The players can change their voices to assume a new role. It may help to look at the pictured scene from the Internet or pamphlet rather than engaging in eye contact initially.

Calling Places of Interest: Parks, Entertainment Sites, Stores for Buying Goods or Clothing, Etc.

1. Secure a picture of the place the child/teen would like to go. If they are a dancer, it could be a dance studio or shop that sells dance clothing and equipment. If they play a sport, it could be a sporting goods store. If they like pets, it could be a pet store. There are many options.
2. Decide what is wanted and write down the sentence(s) to ask the person who answers the phone, or if in person, the clerk.
3. Rehearse the sentence(s).
4. Role-play the scene with the child or teen. Decide on the roles and take turns.
5. Players can change their voice and/or turn around so as not to be seen for the role, if desired.

Text or E-Mail: Communicating Through Text or E-Mail

1. Ask the child or teen to choose a person they know but someone they do not readily speak to. Family members can help them select a cousin, old friend, relative, neighbor, classmate, or someone else.
2. The parent can help establish a connection with that person first and if comfortable can ask that person to reach out to their child via text or e-mail for a reason.
3. Questions related to how they are doing, what is new, what they are doing, how school is going, or another specific question are often best for the initiator to ask.
4. The child/teen should know the text/e-mail is coming soon and can let the parent or facilitator know when they get the text/e-mail if they want help in their reply.

Conversational Tennis: Responding and Initiating in Real-Life Conversations

1. During your encounter with the child/teen, share something about your week in a statement. For example, say, "I had a really hectic day."
2. The child/teen is encouraged to reply if they do not do so automatically.
3. If they do not reply, state the comment again and wait 5 seconds. If they still do not reply, ask them questions such as, "What can you say or ask when someone tells you they had a really hectic day?" If still no response, provide options. "You could ask me what happened?" or "Why was it hectic?" Try it.
4. Provide an answer and encourage the child or teen to say something back. A possibility is, "I hope your day gets better."
5. Redo the short conversation from beginning to end.
6. Some other comments to start a natural conversation may include the following:
    a. I'm not feeling well.
    b. I'm worried about my dog.
    c. I got a new bike.

d. My school cancelled classes this week.
e. I had a problem at the supermarket the other day.
f. My car broke down yesterday.
g. I couldn't get to work the other day.
h. The weather has been nice lately.
i. My cell phone isn't working.
j. My house lost power earlier today, and I wasn't able to use my computer.
k. I like your outfit.
l. I can't wait to go on a vacation.

7. Tell the child/teen that you would like to keep the conversation tennis game going for at least five turns each. Provide options if they don't know what to say, and then redo the conversation in a more fluid manner the second time. It is helpful to write down the sentences for replay.
8. To practice initiations, choose a game (video game, card game, board game, or action game) to play with family and once the game and rules are known, invite someone with whom the child/teen responds but does not typically initiate. Be sure to rehearse and role-play the rules with the child or teen so they know how to give instructions and guide the play. Check https://cardgames.io/ for written rules and demonstrations to some of the most popular games.

CONGRATULATIONS. THE CHILD/TEEN IS BETTER AT SOCIAL PRAGMATIC COMMUNICATION AND READY TO MOVE TO MODULE 3.

References

Altman, I., & Taylor, D. A. (1973). *Social penetration: The development of interpersonal relationships.* Holt, Rinehart & Winston.

American Speech-Language-Hearing Association (ASHA). (2020, December). *Social communication.* https://asha.org/public/speech/development/social-communication/

Amster, B. J., & Klein, E. R. (2018). The impact of perfectionism on stuttering. In B. J. Amster & E. R. Klein (Eds.), *More than fluency: The social, emotional, and cognitive dimensions of stuttering.* Plural Publishing.

Bloodstein, O., & Bernstein Ratner, N. (2008). *A handbook on stuttering* (6th ed.). Thomson-Delmar.

Bögels, S. M., Alden, L., Beidel, D. C., Clark, L. A., Pine, D. S., Stein, M. B., & Voncken, M. (2010), Social anxiety disorder: Questions and answers for the DSM-V. *Depression and Anxiety, 27,* 168–189. https://doi.org/10.1002/da.20670

Boyle, M. P., Milewski, K. M., & Beita-Ell, C. (2018). Disclosure of stuttering and quality of life in people who stutter. *Journal of Fluency Disorders, 58,* 1–10.

Brocklehurst, P. H., Drake, E., & Corley, M. (2015). Perfectionism and stuttering: Findings of an online survey. *Journal of Fluency Disorders, 44*¸ 46–62.

Bunnell, B. E., Mesa, F., & Beidel, D. (2018). A two-session hierarchy for shaping successive approximations of speech in selective mutism: Pilot study of mobile apps and mechanisms of behavior change. *Behavior Therapy, 49,* 966–980.

Burns, D. (1980, November). The perfectionist's script for self-defeat. *Psychology Today,* 34–52.

Cherney, L., Shadden, B., & Coelho, C. (1998). *Analyzing discourse in communicatively impaired adults—Rehabilitation Institute of Chicago*, Aspen.

Crocker, J., Major, B., & Steele, C. (1998). Social stigma. In D. T. Gilbert, S. T. Fiske, & G. Lindzey (Eds.), *The handbook of social psychology* (pp. 89–107). McGraw-Hill.

DeDe, G., & Hoover, E. (2021). Measuring change at the discourse-level following conversation treatment. *Topics in Language Disorders, 41*(1), 5–26.

Devitt, M., & Hanley, R. (2003). Speech acts and pragmatics. *Blackwell guide to philosophy of language.* https://doi.org/10.1016/B0-08-044854-2/04301-7

Essberger, J. (2020). *English club.* https://www.englishclub.com/vocabulary/common-words.htm

Fillmore, C. J. (1979). On fluency. In C. J. Fillmore, D. Kempler, & W. S. Y. Wang (Eds.), *Individual differences in language ability and language behavior* (pp. 85–101). Academic Press.

Franic, D. M., & Bothe, A. K. (2008). Psychometric evaluation of condition-specific instruments used to assess health-related quality of life, attitudes, and related constructs in stuttering. *American Journal of Speech-Language Pathology, 17,* 60–80.

Galbraith, P., Nicksic-Springer, T., & O'Brien, S. (2008, Summer). Building blocks behavior. *Quarterly Newsletter of the Neurobehavior H.O.M.E. Program.*

Goberis, D., Beams, D., Dalpes, M., Abrisch, A., Baca, R., & Yoshinaga-Itano, C. (2012). The missing link in language development: Social communication development. *Seminars in Speech and Language, 33*(4), 297–309.

Iverach, L., Rapee, R. M., Wong, Q. J. J., & Lowe, R. (2017). Maintenance of social anxiety in stuttering: A cognitive-behavioral model. *American Journal of Speech-Language Pathology, 26,* 540–556.

Johnson, M., & Wintgens, A. (2016). *The selective mutism resource manual* (2nd ed.). Speechmark Publishing.

Klein, E. R., Armstrong, S. L., Gordon, J., Kennedy, D., Satko, C., & Shipon-Blum, E. (2018). *Expanding receptive and expressive skills through stories: Language formulation in children with selective mutism and other communication needs.* Plural Publishing.

Klein, E. R., Armstrong, S. L., & Shipon-Blum, E. (2013). Assessing spoken language competence in children with selective mutism: Using parents as test presenters. *Communication Disorders Quarterly, 34*(3), 184–195. https://journals.sagepub.com/doi/10.1177/1525740112455053

Laugeson, E. A. (2017). *PEERS for young adults.* Routledge.

Lichtwarck-Aschoff, A., & Rooji, M. M. J. W. (2019). Are changes in children's communication patterns predictive of treatment outcomes for children with anxiety? *Clinical Psychology & Psychotherapy, 26*(5), 572–585. https://doi.org/10.1002/cpp.2383

Mancinelli, J. M. (2018). A perspective on stuttering in the social context. In B. J. Amster & E. R. Klein (Eds.), *More than fluency: The social, emotional, and cognitive dimensions of stuttering.* Plural Publishing.

Mancinelli, J. M. (2019). The effects of self-disclosure on the conversational interaction between a person who stutters and a normally fluent speaker. *Journal of Fluency Disorders, 59,* 1–20.

McInnes, A., Fung, D., Manassis, K., Fiksenbaum, L., & Tannock, R. (2004). Narrative skills in children with selective mutism: An exploratory study. *American Journal of Speech-Language Pathology, 13*(4), 304–315. https://doi.org/10.1044/1058-0360(2004/031

Melero, S., Morales, A., Espada, J. P., Fernández-Martinez, & Orgilés, M. (2020). How does perfectionism influence the development of psychological strengths and difficulties in children? *International Journal of Environmental Research and Public Health,* 17(11), 4081. https://doi.org/10.3390/ijerph17114081

Nippold, M. A., Frantz-Kaspar, M. W., Cramond, P. M., Kirk, C., Hayward-Mayhew, C., & MacKinnon, M. (2014). Conversational and narrative speaking in adolescents: Examining the use of complex syntax. *Journal of Speech, Language, and Hearing Research, 57,* 876– 886.

Oerbeck, B., Stein, M. B., Wentzel-Larsen, T., Langsrud, O., & Kristense, H. (2014). A randomized controlled trial of a home and school-based intervention for selective mutism—Defocused communication and behavioural techniques. *Child and Adolescent Mental Health, 19*(3), 192–198.

Russell, R. L. (2007). Social communication impairments: Pragmatics. *Pediatric Clinics of North America, 54*(3), 483–506. https://doi.org/10.1016/j.pcl.2007.02.016

Searle, J. R. (1975), Speech acts and recent linguistics. *Annals of the New York Academy of Sciences, 263*, 27–38. https://doi.org/10.1111/j.1749-6632.1975.tb41567.x

Sisskin, V. (2018). Avoidance reduction therapy for stuttering. In B. J. Amster & E. R. Klein (Eds.), *More than fluency: The social, emotional, and cognitive dimensions of stuttering.* Plural Publishing.

Smith, A., & Kelly, E. (1997). Stuttering: A dynamic multifactorial model. In R. Curlee & G. Siegel (Eds.), *Nature and treatment of stuttering: New directions* (2nd ed.). Allyn & Bacon.

Snyder, G., Williams, M. G., Adams, C., & Blanchet, P. (2020). The effects of different sources of stuttering disclosure on the perceptions of a child who stutters. *Language, Speech, and Hearing Service in Schools, 51*, 741–760.

Starkweather, C. W. (1987). *Fluency and stuttering.* Prentice Hall.

Ukrainetz, T. A. (2015). Improving reading comprehension: More than meets the eye. In. T. A. Ukrainetz (Ed.), *School-age language intervention: Evidence-based practices* (pp. 565– 607). Pro-Ed.

Vassilopoulos, S. P., & Banerjee, R. (2010). Social interaction anxiety and the discounting of positive interpersonal events. *Behavioural and Cognitive Psychotherapy, 38*, 597–609.

Voncken, M. J., & Bögels, S. M. (2008). Social performance deficits in social anxiety disorder: Reality during conversation and biased perception during speech. *Journal of Anxiety Disorders, 22*(8), 1384–1392. https://doi.org/10.1016/j.janxdis.2008.02.001

Winner, M. G. (2007). *Thinking about you thinking about me* (2nd ed.). Think Social Publishing.

Yaruss, J. S., & Quesal, R. W. (2006). Overall Assessment of the Speaker's Experience of Stuttering (OASES): Documenting multiple outcomes in stuttering treatment. *Journal of Fluency Disorders, 31*, 90–115.

Appendix 2–A

SUGGESTIONS FOR FACILITATING ACTIVITIES FOR CHILDREN AND TEENS WITH SELECTIVE MUTISM

Getting the Voice Started in Context

Children or teens with selective mutism may be hesitant to speak initially, especially with individuals with whom they are not familiar. Since they have completed Module 1, they can use their voice for making sounds, saying words, and saying sentences. If *initiating voice* is challenging for an activity, remind the child or teen to use the humming [m] sound for greater ease with voice initiation. This method allows voice to be directed through the nose (as a nasal sound). To get started, a short humming sound with the letter "m" will help the vocal cords vibrate and make sound. Once the humming sound is generated in an almost inaudible manner, change it to the first sound in the word that the child or teens wants to say. The [h] sound can also be used to initiate airflow for greater ease with voice initiation. Visual imagery can also help the child/teen think of related words to say. Ask the child/teen to visualize what the object or action looks like and think of related items and words.

Expanding Speech to New Communication Partners

If the online version of this program is used, the child/teen can turn the video off while speaking, initially. It may also help to pair the child/teen with someone with whom they speak more readily (such as a parent or friend) and for the facilitator to be the other person listening while slowly sharing a few sentences with the parent or friend who has joined the conversation. A *fading-in or sliding-in approach* (Johnson & Wintgens, 2016) can help because the parent/friend is the person with whom the child or teen has a speaking relationship. For the sliding-in process, the facilitator appears busy with something while the child/teen and parent/friend engage in the activity. The facilitator joins in periodically saying a sentence. This person makes a positive comment about what the child/teen and parent/friend are doing. In a nonchalant way, the two-way conversation can expand to all three people after a few encounters.

Speaking in the school setting is often most difficult due to expectations and performance-related anxiety. It can be beneficial to include a keyworker from the school (a teacher, therapist, or another helper such as a parent or sibling with whom the child speaks). The sliding-in approach (Johnson & Wintgens, 2016) can help because the keyworker is usually a person with whom the child or teen has a relationship. The keyworker and the child/teen can engage in conversation during an art activity or while playing a board game.

- For the sliding-in process, the third, less familiar person, enters the space where the keyworker and child/teen are playing or working.
- The third person acts busy with something at a distance and then leaves the space.

- Shortly afterward, that third less familiar person returns and walks to another space in the room for a few minutes and then walks closer to the keyworker and child/teen.
- This person makes a positive comment about what the child/teen and keyworker are doing but does not address the child/teen directly.
- In a nonchalant way, the two-way conversation with the keyworker can extend to all three people after several encounters. The third person has joined the activity.
- After the child or teen becomes more comfortable with the third person, the keyworker can slowly be phased out.

Using Writing for Speaking

Children with selective mutism have been found to produce shorter, simpler narratives with less details than age-matched peers in both home and clinic settings. They produce fewer clauses, and their syntactic skills can be less well-developed (Klein et al., 2013; McInnes et al., 2004). Generating new sentences can require assistance, especially if trying to stay on topic. The child/teen can begin by *writing a sentence and then reading it* aloud if helpful. This is useful for someone who is reluctant to speak spontaneously and needs time to think of what to say. They can also dictate their sentence into a smartphone or recording device and play it back for the facilitator to hear.

The more challenging the task, the less familiar the environment, and the more people involved, the greater the avoidance. The child/teen with selective mutism generally avoids asking for things that are needed when in uncomfortable settings. This can present problems accomplishing tasks correctly. To ask questions if something is unclear, the child/teen can write their question and read it aloud so that their focus is on the paper with less pressure for spontaneous speech.

Responsiveness With Defocused Communication

Since the expectation to speak can increase fear, it is important not to react when hearing a child or teen read their part aloud, even though a tendency to comment with excitement when hearing the child or teen speak is common. Continue *listening without reacting* to the child/teen's speaking parts even if their voice is quiet but still audible (Johnson & Wintgens, 2016). A nonchalant demeanor is best.

Direct questions can feel uncomfortable or even threatening to some. To help increase comfort when answering or asking questions, try using a barrier (trifold poster board or file folders) placed in between the two speakers. The child/teen can also turn to the side or move farther away from the other person to increase comfort initially.

Approximately 65% of children with selective mutism have been identified as meeting diagnostic criteria for social anxiety disorder (Bögels et al., 2010). *Defocused communication* has been found to help alleviate anxiety for children with selective mutism and can be incorporated into activities. Research has found that the following strategies can reduce anxiety for those with selective mutism: (1) reducing eye contact and focusing on materials, (2) looking around slightly when speaking, (3) sitting next to the child/teen instead of across from them, (4) talking aloud to oneself about what is happening as if thinking out loud, and (5) giving them time to respond instead of responding for them (Oerbeck et al., 2014).

Responsiveness With Modified Question Types

Children with selective mutism have difficulty responding to questions because questions put them "on the spot" with a direct request for speech. They are more likely to respond to yes-no type questions than *wh-* questions; however, yes-no questions do not usually support an interactive dialogue or require expanded responses. The most challenging task is often initiating questions, especially with people who are less familiar. At times, using pictures or objects can help foster dialogue as it makes responses more contextual.

There are a few things that can make the progression from answering questions to initiating them a bit easier. It is easier to accept head nods for yes-no questions than answering yes or no verbally. However, this is not preferred. The child/teen often finds it easier to write their answers and then read them, but that takes time. Changing a *wh-* question to a choice question is another helpful strategy to help the child/teen respond. Before changing the question, give the child/teen time to think of an answer. If they do not answer, wait about 5 seconds and ask again.

Keep eye contact to a minimum while waiting. After asking a second time, and still without a reply, ask once again and wait another 5 seconds. If there is still no reply, offer some logical choices. For example, if you asked, "When do you think people should be able to drive a car?" and no response is given after two attempts, ask the question once more and give choices by adding "16 years old, 18 years old, or some other age?" If still no reply, change to a yes-no question such as, "Do you think people should be able to drive when they are 16 years old?" If the child/teen nods for an answer, ask, "Is that yes or no?" They are more likely to provide a yes or no response verbally when asked that way. This hierarchy is often beneficial and supports *modifying question types* (Klein et al., 2018). Computer-based apps or games are also beneficial in helping children ask and answer open-ended *wh-* questions. Games and apps inhibit the individual's impulse to remain silent when uncomfortable (Bunnell et al., 2018).

Giving Praise

When working with children or teens who have selective mutism, it is best to focus on materials in view and minimize direct face-to-face eye contact initially. During any activity, it is a good idea to *give brief labeled praise*. This is praise that is specific and includes the following:

- *Praise* an action.
- *Reflect* on a situation by stating what is happening.
- *Imitate* appropriate skills and play.
- *Describe* appropriate behavior.
- Show moderated *Enthusiasm*.

The following link provides explanations and examples for the acronym PRIDE (Galbraith et al., 2008): http://static1.1.sqspcdn.com/static/f/1057879/14796377/1319510543780/ PRIDE+handout.pdf?token=6OAiUF8PIzzKuxAlxvS40yfsJJE%3D

Identifying Levels of Communication Difficulty

The facilitator may use a "1 to 10" graph to learn more about how the child/teen feels about accomplishing challenging tasks. On the graph, write the numbers 1 to 10 from left to right.

Under the number "1" draw a calm, happy-looking face and the words "Very easy" or "Yes, absolutely" and under the number "10" draw a worried or sad face and the words "Very hard" or "No way." Then say, *"On a scale from 1 to 10, with 1 being very easy and 10 being very difficult or hard, how is it for you to ___________ (i.e., 'say hi to ___________ in your class?')."* If applicable, ask the child/teen what they think could be done to help make it easier. If they do not know, provide some ideas such as writing down what to say and reading it, texting it, and then saying it, or role-playing it, etc. Remind the child/teen that avoiding the task makes the skill more challenging but that trying small steps leads to progress.

Contributing to a Conversation

The most difficult part of staying on topic for someone with selective mutism is fighting the urge to stay silent. According to Lichtwarck-Aschoff and van Rooji (2019), breaking rigid patterns of communication, such as only answering questions but not asking questions, is important to improving interactions. During turn-taking in conversations, both responding and initiating are predictive of more positive social outcomes. Initiating topics is often more difficult.

The child/teen can learn to *contribute to a conversation* by asking the same questions that were asked of them. For children and teens with selective mutism who do not respond or initiate, the facilitator is encouraged to provide sentences for the child or teen to repeat. They can write the sentences for practice first. The child or teen can practice adding to a conversation by repeating what the facilitator says and then do it on their own.

Expanding Sentence Complexity and Maintaining the Conversation

Conversations can be challenging (Johnson & Wintgens, 2016). Texting or instant messaging may be an easier way to start if the child or teen uses a smartphone. If the child/teen uses single-word answers, encourage them to *add more words* by including connector words such as *"for," "and," "but," "or," "so,"* and *"because"* to expand their sentences. They can also start a new sentence with something about themself by using the word, "I." Comments or questions can be used to keep an interaction going. Some include the following:

- *"That's cool!"*
- *"Oh no!"*
- *"Awesome."*
- *"Great!"*
- *"Interesting."*
- *"What else happened?"*
- *"When did that happen?"*
- *"What are you gonna do about it?"*
- *"I hope it works out for you."*

When leaving the conversation, it is fine to say the following:

- *"I have to go now."*
- *"Talk to ya later."*
- *"Bye."*
- *"See ya."*

After a conversation has taken place, review it with the child/teen. To increase awareness about what happened in the dialogue, reenact it. This can be done (to some extent) from memory or by redoing a script if it was written or taped. During initial sessions, it is common for the child/teen with selective mutism to only answer the facilitator's questions with a word or short phrase and say no more. The conversation ends quickly. It can be helpful to replay the scene using *wh-*questions instead of Yes-No questions. The facilitator can also *say sentences to expand conversational skills* for the child/teen to repeat, thereby learning how to include them in a conversation. This can support those same skills in real-life situations with a store clerk, restaurant server, nurse, doctor, teacher, friend's parent, or other individuals.

Gaining Comfort in Anxiety-Producing Situations

As the child/teen moves into more realistic and challenging speaking situations, a few recommended strategies can be used as scaffolds to reduce anxiety (Klein et al., 2018). These include the following:

- Keep a calm and less assertive demeanor when interacting with the child/teen as being overly exuberant can increase anxiety.
- Minimalize expectations for eye contact and focus on the items at hand for greater comfort.
- Try to limit use of the words "talk" and "speak." Rather use the terms, "use your voice" or "use your words."
- Allow the child/teen to speak into a recorder and bring the device to the facilitator to hear or have the child/teen speak to a familiar person in front of the facilitator, allowing their voice to be overheard. These are encouraging steps toward more direct and audible speech with new people.
- Do not attempt to coerce the child to speak. Be sure to get the child/teen's approval to share any audio or videotapes of them with others.

Changing One Thing at a Time

Experience and exposure are important to being comfortable having a conversation in new situations or with people who are less familiar. As the child or teen gains skills and moves toward having spontaneous conversations, it is crucial that the facilitator does not expect too much too fast. Progression requires changing one thing at a time so as not to overwhelm the child/teen. If they can have a chat with the facilitator in one setting and all seems to be going well, do not assume they can do the same with their teacher at school or with a friend at that friend's house. In those scenarios, the place, person, or activity may have changed.

- When moving toward new experiences speaking, remember the rule of *changing only one thing at a time*. Consider (1) the people whom they encounter, (2) the place of the encounters, and (3) the activities they are to engage in. Therefore, if the child/teen is going to do a new activity they have not done before, keep the people and place the same. Only change the activity. The same is true for any of the three considerations.
- Remember that any communication is better than no communication. Audible whispering or writing can be acceptable in new encounters initially.
- Refrain from putting too much pressure on the child/teen but work toward new goals each session. Questioning strategies, moving from open-ended, *wh-* questions to responding to choices can be helpful in scaffolding responses at the start of a new task.

Appendix 2–B

SUGGESTIONS FOR FACILITATING ACTIVITIES FOR CHILDREN AND TEENS WHO STUTTER

Putting the Stutter Where It Belongs

When working with a child or teen who stutters, here are some things to think about and talk about. Using a phrase *fight to make it right* addresses the issue of avoidance, that is *avoiding* avoidance, whereas using a phrase *put the stutter where it belongs* facilitates open stuttering or stuttering freely with greater self-acceptance (Sisskin, 2018). The following questions can be used to address the affective, behavioral, and cognitive (ABC) aspects of stuttering as well as helping the child/teen to connect with the physiological sensations associated with their stuttering (Amster & Klein, 2018; Mancinelli, 2018, 2019). This facilitates the development of an understanding that their stuttering is multidimensional (Bloodstein & Bernstein Ratner, 2008; Smith & Kelly, 1997). Here are some questions that can be posed to address the ABCs. The facilitator can expand on topics by asking some or all of the following questions:

- *How does it feel when you say a word and stutter on it?*
- *Do you feel any tension anywhere in or on your body when you say the word? If you do, where is it?*
- *Do you have any tools or strategies that you can use to produce it again but without the tension? If so, try saying the word again using those tools.*
- If the child/teen stuttered when they said the word, ask them, *Did you put the stutter where it belongs or did you fight to make it right? Does it feel more comfortable to fight to make it right or to put the stutter where it belongs?*
- *Do you listen to your communication partner when they are taking a turn?*
- *What do you think about when you are talking?*
- *Does your speech change based on the person or topic you are discussing?*
- *Give the child/teen the option to reboot and say it again!*

Keep in mind that an important element in the treatment of stuttering with children and teens is to reduce their negative perception about themselves as communicator and to "de-awfulize" stuttering. It helps the individual develop self-efficacy and self-agency as a communicator.

Building Confidence

Building confidence as an effective communicator is important for the child or teen who stutters even if their speech may not be as fluent as they would like. They also need to feel free to stutter openly without concentrated attention to the listener's response to their speech (Iverach et al., 2017; Mancinelli, 2018). It is important to foster the willingness and ability to cope with stuttering. Individuals who are highly perfectionistic may have difficulty coping.

Children and teens who have perfectionistic tendencies for speech often live with unrealistic personal standards, which can lead to feelings of lower self-esteem (Burns, 1980). For the individual who stutters, these tendencies "to get it right" can inhibit them from sharing information or asking for clarification. Fear of stuttering is at the root of this inhibition, that is, they may be focusing on not stuttering instead of getting and/or sharing information.

Brocklehurst, Drake, and Corley (2015) found that people who stutter were more concerned about making mistakes (doubts about actions) on the Frost Multidimensional Perfectionism Scale. For those who have heightened concerns about making a mistake, worries can prevent the child or teen from asking questions or getting information they need in the classroom about assignments, project due dates, and so on. Here are some things to think about when working with the child/teen who stutters.

- Start with one word at a time and then move on to making a sentence with that word. If the child or teen is using *stuttering modification techniques* or *fluency shaping techniques* in treatment, prompt them as necessary. This may include using light bounces to stutter more easily to release tension and/or using easy onset on words starting with vowels, light articulatory contacts with consonants, continuous voicing technique, and/or other strategies that are part of the individual's therapeutic plan.

Taking Turns

When we have conversations with other people, we each have a turn to speak. Sometimes we take that turn, and sometimes we do not. Some people talk a lot and other people talk a little, and that is okay. Reading aloud is another way to practice using speech. For example, reading a speech, reciting a poem, or giving a presentation are some ways that speech and reading are connected. *Take turns* reading and filling in the blanks to create a short conversation. When two people are talking to each other, the most important thing to remember is not "how do I sound" but "are my sounds telling the other person what I want them to know?"

- In this activity, encourage the child to use fluency enhancing techniques such as easy onset on words starting with vowels, light articulatory contacts with consonants, and/or other strategies that are part of the individual's therapeutic plan.
- Ask, *"Were you thinking about me listening to you while you were taking your turn? If so, tell me about that. Do you ever think about the listener while taking your turn in a conversation?"*

Let the child or teen know that as Communicator-in-Chief, they make their own decisions about their speech and their message. Ask the child or teen what kind of decisions they are making during a conversation with another person. For example, are they thinking about conveying their message, their speech fluency, how to avoid stuttering, or how to stutter more openly and freely by putting the stutter where it belongs?

Feeling Free to Stutter

One of the goals of this program is to develop the child/teen's confidence as an effective communicator in a conversational context about varied topics. However, speech onset can be problematic for a person who stutters because the vocal folds are moving from a resting position (Starkweather, 1987). Laryngeal blocks can occur and that can spiral into greater dysfluency, silence, and further reinforcement of the notion that the individual is unable to communicate without stuttering. It can be helpful to contrast fluent speech from blocks, prolongations, or repetitions. Remind the child/teen that easy onset, continuous voicing, and stuttering easily are available tools to enhance fluency. Try pseudostuttering to gain a clearer understanding of what the child/teen does when they stutter. This can help identify differences during speech and provide information about how to move toward a more relaxed state of speaking. Remind the child/teen to use stuttering modification techniques or fluency-shaping techniques that they are familiar with. While the child or teen is talking, the focus is on facilitating easier stuttering.

- Encourage the child/teen to *feel free to stutter* to reduce their tendency to control their stuttering. Tell them to let their words fly free as a kite! It is important to remember that stuttering is very idiosyncratic, so individuals can be at different stages in their acceptance of their stuttering as well as their ability to use fluency enhancing techniques. This means that the facilitator is free to inject desensitization techniques, cognitive restructuring, and so on, at any time, based on the clinical presentation of the client. Use the following questions to address the cognitive and affective aspects of stuttering:
  - ☐ *How did it feel to stutter freely?*
  - ☐ *How did it feel when you were trying to avoid your stuttering?*
  - ☐ *Were you thinking about your speech when you were asking for clarification or giving directions?*
  - ☐ *Were you using any of your tools to help you? Which ones?*
  - ☐ *Talk about "letting your words fly."*

Facilitating Desensitization

For people who stutter, any conversational interaction can be perceived as a primary threat (Crocker et al., 1998). Therefore, avoiding those interactions decreases anxiety around stuttering, possible listener reactions, and feelings of stigmatization. In the case of children and teens who stutter, the clinician can use this activity to focus on stuttering freely, stuttering more easily, or putting the stutter where it belongs during the conversation. This *facilitates desensitization*, getting in touch with their stuttering and not fearing it, and learning *how* to stutter more easily. The ultimate goal, of course, is self-acceptance as an effective communicator who stutters, and not a stutterer who cannot communicate. The following questions are often beneficial to reflect on thoughts and experiences:

- *How do you feel about asking and answering questions?*
- *What are you thinking about when someone asks you a question?*
- *What are you thinking about when you want to ask someone a question?*

- *Who do you feel most comfortable speaking to? Least comfortable?*
- *Where are you most comfortable speaking? Why?*
- *When do you feel most comfortable speaking to others? Why?*
- *Why do you feel comfortable speaking sometimes and not as comfortable at other times? Do these places have anything in common?*
- *How does talking to others change based on the type of talking that you are doing?*
- *Are you more comfortable giving a speech, talking to a parent, or talking to a friend?*

Anticipating Listeners' Reactions

Facilitate a discussion around the issue of the *listener's reactions to stuttering*, level of comfort under each condition, and self-perceptions of stuttering. Engage in a discussion given the following questions:

- *Are you concerned about a listener's reactions during a conversation?*
- *How would you rate your speech fluency when attention is not focused on you?*
- *Can you stutter freely? Do you put the stutter where it belongs, or do you fight to make it right?*
- *How do you feel when it is your turn to speak?*
- *Are you thinking about how your speech sounds when it was your turn, or just sending the message?*
- *Talk about feelings and thoughts during the activities.*

Varying Types of Talk

Conversational role-plays can be used to examine, expand, and/or develop social uses of language for children and teens who stutter. A speaker's "fluency competence" can be measured by looking at four features: the ability to talk at length with limited pauses (*talkativeness*), the ability to talk in coherent and syntactically complex sentences (*succinctness*), the ability to speak on a variety of topics (*flexibility*), and the ability to be creative and imaginative with language (*creativity*) (Fillmore, 1979). Starkweather (1987) augmented Fillmore's four elements by adding continuity (*keeping sounds and words connected*), rate of speech, rhythm (*prosodic patterns within a message*), and effort (*the amount of energy the speaker expends when talking*). It is also possible to work on the social aspects of communication from a speech acts perspective (Searle, 1975). Once the child or teen completes a conversation, review the following list and see how many of those *types of talk* were included in the conversation:

1. *Greetings/hello/opening a conversation*
2. *Leaving/goodbyes/closing a conversation*
3. *Thanking/showing appreciation*
4. *Commenting or complimenting*
5. *Apologizing*

6. *Requesting clarification or information*
7. *Stating a problem or making an excuse*
8. *Making a complaint or complaining*
9. *Asking for help or offering help*
10. *Providing information*

The added dimension of speech fluency can be woven into the session.

Disclosing Stuttering

Disclosure about stuttering may be another consideration as it has been found to reduce individuals' attempts to control their stuttering. According to Boyle, Milewski, and Beita-Ell (2018), disclosure of stuttering has been related to increased quality of life. A discussion about disclosing one's stuttering may be helpful. In research by Snyder, Williams, Adams, and Blanchet (2020), disclosure had benefits for children. Results indicated that self-disclosure (via video) by a 12-year-old boy had a positive effect on the child's perceptions from more than 200 young adults who viewed the video. The boy's personal characteristics were identified as being more calm (than nervous), more relaxed (than tense), more confident (than insecure), more friendly (than unfriendly), more outgoing (than shy), more competent (than incompetent), and more approachable (than unapproachable) to a statistically significant degree from disclosing his stuttering. Therefore, practicing ways to include statements about being a person who stutters or mentioning something about one's stuttering may be worthwhile.

The Overall Assessment of the Speaker's Experience of Stuttering (OASES) (Yaruss & Quesal, 2006) may be useful for children (7 to 12 years old) or teens (13 to 17 years old). This measure is recommended as it includes areas regarding *general information about the speaker's perception of stuttering, reactions to stuttering, difficulties with communication in daily situations,* and *overall impact of quality of life.* This reliable and valid measure can help gauge progress at intervals throughout the program (Franic & Bothe, 2008).

Module 3

ROLE-PLAY SIMULATIONS FOR CONVERSATION

Background Information

Module 3 is uniquely designed to engage individuals in daily acts of communication. In Modules 1 and 2, we guide individuals with selective mutism and stuttering from the initial stages of using and manipulating their voices to the social pragmatic skills of conversation through games. The learned skills are now practiced via role-plays to simulate various daily activities where they speak at home, in school, and in public settings.

Individuals with selective mutism and stuttering may feel uncomfortable or anxious in daily activities, derailing idea generation, complex sentence formation, and conversational fluency for different purposes. Therefore, Module 3 will improve their conversational skills, so the anxiety no longer impedes performance.

Theoretical Framework

Our primary methodology for the role-plays loosely follows the work of Paul Heinrich (2018). In his work, he lays out the four sections typically needed to establish a scenario before walking into the role-playing activity. These are *Characterization*, "Who am I?"; *History*, "What has brought me to this moment?"; *Anticipated shape of the drama*, "What am I walking into?"; and *Educational considerations*, "What are we hoping to achieve through this interaction?"

The scenarios we created for the role-play experiences were drawn from the 17 scenarios in the validated Selective Mutism Questionnaire (SMQ) (Bergman et al., 2008; https://www.oxfordclinicalpsych.com/view/10.1093/med:psych/9780195391527.001.0001/med-9780195391527-interactive-pdf-002.pdf).

The 17 corresponding role-play activities reflect speaking situations in school, at home, and in public settings. This questionnaire, while specific to selective mutism, is appropriate as a guide for speaking situations with communication and may be applied to those who stutter as they relate to frequency of speaking in different situations with perceived degree of interference in those settings.

Each of the 17 role-play activities include two variations, one that incorporates more dialogue and another with less. As part of the experience, we identified 15 possible cognitive distortions or distorted thinking related to the communication scenarios. Cognitive distortions are noted to be intrinsic to the development and maintenance of anxiety-related thoughts (Kaplan et al., 2017). Cognitive distortions are errors in thinking based on how individuals process situations that generally upset them in school and other settings. This kind of thinking may seem rational and accurate to someone who struggles with communication difficulties. Believing that negative consequences will ensue from communicative interactions can make interacting with others more difficult and should be challenged.

In each of the 17 role-play situations, we present two probable cognitive distortions and alternative considerations. All 15 cognitive distortions from the Cognitive Distortions Questionnaire (CD-Quest) (Kaplan et al., 2017) appear at least once so that the facilitator and client can contemplate a new way to think about a situation that may be challenging. This measure developed at the Trial-Based Cognitive Therapy Institute is psychometrically reliable and valid. It is the most comprehensive, evidence-based assessment of cognitive distortions available today.

Using the SMQ as a Guide for Activity Selection and Tracking Progress

To begin, download the SMQ form at the following link: https://www.oxfordclinicalpsych.com/view/10.1093/med:psych/9780195391527.001.0001/med-9780195391527-interactive-pdf-002.pdf

There are 23 items on the questionnaire. The first 17 relate to frequency of speaking in the three situations. The last six items relate to degree of interference and distress felt. The information obtained from this form can be used as a guide for activity selection and for tracking progress over time.

To implement, follow these instructions. Tell the child or teen the following:

- *I am going to ask you a total of 17 questions that relate to speaking in school, at home, and in social situations outside of school.*
- *You can choose any one of the situations to start.*
- *For each question I ask you, you can select "Almost Always," "Often," "Seldom," or "Never." You can say, point to, or circle your answer.*
  - □ The facilitator will need to say the statement with a change in pronouns so that Item/Scenario 5, "When appropriate, my child speaks to most teachers or staff at school" becomes *"When appropriate, I speak to most teachers or staff at school."* Then as facilitator, follows the statement with *Is that "Almost Always," "Often," "Seldom," or "Never"?*
- *You'll choose the best fit for how it is NOW, and then I will ask you again for how you WANT IT TO BE. You may choose SELDOM for Item/Scenario 3, "When called on by my teacher, I answer" and when asked about how you want it to be, your answer may become OFTEN. It is totally up to you.*

NOW	WANT TO BE
Almost Always	Almost Always
Often	Often
Seldom	Seldom
Almost Never	Almost Never

- Using the information from the child or teen, start with the item/scenario that they want to move up one level (e.g., going from "Often" to "Always" or from "Seldom" to "Often" and consider working on that to begin in Module 3.

Role-Play Structure

The following sections present the elements that comprise each scenario and two accompanying situations.

Facilitator

The facilitator is the person who is coaching the role-play. The facilitator can pause the role- play, ask questions, or make suggestions at any time. Often, the facilitator is a clinician, typically a speech-language pathologist, psychologist, counselor, parent, or teacher.

Player

Anyone participating in the role-play is a "player." The facilitator may participate in this way if more players are needed in the activity.

Scenario

The scenario is the overall circumstance for each role-play activity. There are 17 scenarios in this module, which correspond to the 17 scenarios in the SMQ (Bergman et al., 2008). There are six scenarios that take place at school, six that take place in the home or with family, and five that take place in other social settings with others outside school and home.

Personal Stories

Each scenario begins with a recollection contributed by a real person who had communication challenges. These descriptions include some moments that will provide insight into how others experience the scenario. The players may be able to relate to some of these thoughts.

Please note, we edited the names and recollections to protect anonymity but preserved the intended meaning.

In Preparation for the Role-Play

This section provides prompts to create personalized material that may be useful in conversation during the role-play. It can be helpful for the players to write down thoughts about a topic in advance and refer to them when needed once the role-play activity begins.

Role-Play/Activity

This section begins with background information about the people and circumstances leading up to the moment to be acted out. This is followed by a step-by-step guide for facilitating the role-play activity. The facilitator can give the numbered instructions one at a time and allow the players to perform each step.

Roles

The role is the character or person that the player is performing within the role-play. Players may choose to play themselves. Alternatively, players may opt to select a role at the end of this module, using the photo cards provided. Players or facilitators are free to swap or change roles if performing the role-play more than once. If an activity has more roles than there are players, it is possible for one player to play more than one role. For this, we recommend holding up the photo card to indicate which role is speaking. If the activity is being done virtually (online or via teletherapy), the facilitator and/or players can switch off their video(s) and set the background as the photo card of their choice. Please note that all genders, pronouns, and names can be changed, and parent or caregiver titles may be substituted.

Situations

At a certain point, each role-play branches into two potential situations, based on either a choice by the main player or the actions of a supporting player. It is best to do both situations for practice, but the facilitator and player can pick which situation they want to perform first. Alternatively, the facilitator and player with advanced role-play skills could do an open improvisation instead of continuing with the situations provided. The facilitator and player could also create their own alternative situation and write an outline or script to follow before enacting it.

Reflections

At the end of each role-play, we included a few questions to prompt discussion. Additional questions to consider include the following:

- *"What would you have liked to happen?"*
- *"Tell me what you're thinking since we did the role play?"*
- *"What do you wish you had done?"*
- *"If you could have changed anything, what would it have been?"*
- *"Why do you think that?"*

Cognitive Distortions

For each scenario, we included two cognitive distortions that may arise in the role-play activity. These are offered as a potential jumping-off point for discussion following the role-play activity. It may be that this feedback session could result in a proposal to repeat the role-play exercise using different choices or behaviors.

For the Facilitator

The facilitator takes responsibility for coaching the role-play and must stay focused for the duration of the activity. Before we start our situational role-play activities, we have a few suggestions.

Tips. These role-plays are a good opportunity to employ skills developed in Modules 1 and 2. If a player gets stuck, offering one of the following prompts provides a previously practiced task to move the dialogue forward:

- Hum to feel vibration on your face and nose to "get the voice motor running."
- Speak with varied pitch and intonation.
- Speak in different volumes throughout the scene: pick a moment to be loud, a moment to be soft, and a moment to be somewhere in between.
- Start a sentence with one of the following phrases:
  - ☐ *"I want . . . "* (Stating your needs)
  - ☐ *"I think you should . . . "* (Giving commands)
  - ☐ *"I feel . . . "* (Expressing your feelings)
  - ☐ *"Me and you . . . "* (Interacting with others)
  - ☐ *"Tell me why . . . "* (Asking questions)
  - ☐ *"I've got something to tell you . . . "* (Sharing information with others)
- Write down some things to say and incorporate them into the next run of the role-play
- Draw a picture or locate an image from somewhere else that might help you express yourself in this activity
- Use gestures with your hands, face, or body to express yourself with body language
- Ask a *wh-* question that applies (who, what, where, when, why, or how)
- Do any of the following formats apply to this scenario:
  - ☐ Greetings/hello
  - ☐ Leaving/goodbye
  - ☐ Thank you
  - ☐ Complimenting
  - ☐ Apologizing
  - ☐ Requesting clarification
  - ☐ Stating a problem or making an excuse
  - ☐ Making a complaint
  - ☐ Asking for help/assistance
  - ☐ Providing information
- Can you use one of these skills for spontaneous conversation: listening, questioning, storytelling, commenting, sharing information, complimenting, agreeing, and disagreeing?
- Think about what you are doing and what you want to accomplish.
- Think of the point you want to get across, not just the words.
- Refer to the Social Communication Skills Pragmatics Checklist (Module 2, Table 2–1).

For the Player

It is not always easy to communicate, especially with people you do not know well or when you are in unfamiliar situations. In these cases, it can be hard to know what to say. There could be many reasons for this, such as uncertainty over what is being discussed, worry about another person's reactions, or feeling like you do not belong. We set up role-play simulations for you to practice to gain comfort with your daily communication skills. These activities build on the skills developed in Module 1, which developed greater awareness of how sound is made and how we use sound and vocal vibrations to talk, and Module 2, which introduced specific techniques about speech acts and how we use words and language to interact and keep a conversation going. You will be asked to play yourself or play a new role, so you can bring out your personality and allow parts of you, that you have been afraid to let other people see, emerge. You can redo the role-play simulation a second time and make the flow better.

Tips. For many of us who want to communicate, we may feel we have to do it right, and we feel like we are performing and do not want to make a mistake or be embarrassed. According to Matt Abrahams (2016), when you talk, there is no right way. Therefore, look at communicating as something like playing or acting. You might say to yourself, "Hey this is me, feeling nervous. Remember, this is normal, and people don't analyze every word I am saying." Sometimes we do not want to say too much because we are nervous about saying the wrong thing. It is not unusual to hear somebody say "Hi" or "Bye" or just wave without further interaction, but you could say more. Add a few more words. Instead of just saying "Hi," add your name and provide more information like, "Hi I'm Lenny. I came here with a friend and I don't know anyone here." A lot of people shut down and hide from others when they feel nervous or threatened. At any point, it is OK if you feel nervous, want to stop paying attention, and get away from the activity or the people. In doing these situational role-playing activities, you will have a chance to act and try out different roles. One of the first things to do is figure out the role you want to play. Keep in mind that when playing a role with another person, that other person may not be someone you would like to spend time with. Not all people you know are people you would want to hang out with.

Realizing who you enjoy being with is of great value and can help you learn about what is important to you. Nevertheless, in real life we often have to speak up to make our needs known, gather information, or help ourselves, regardless of who we are speaking to.

Some of these stories and characters may feel familiar to you, while others may be different from your real-life experiences. Either way, commit to the role-play and include in your feedback how you and your character compare or contrast. We hope you find this to be an exciting opportunity that leads you toward easier communication and conversation.

Scenario 1: Talking to General Peers at School

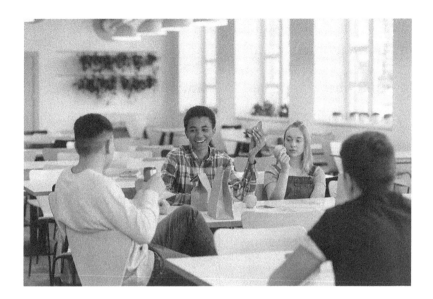

Josie's Story

"During lunch period, I sit near my brother and his friends who I know won't pay attention to me. I avoid situations where I am pressured to speak. I really like video games and know a lot about them, but when someone brings it up, I am scared to go with the urge to say something. I'm always afraid of sounding awkward when I talk. I might benefit from listening to a conversation and hearing what other people are saying—maybe they make mistakes when they speak too. But I do not want them to notice me and then prompt me to respond. So, I stay quiet and don't pay attention to any of them. I know that staying quiet all the time keeps me alone, without friends at school and that bothers me."

In Preparation for the Role-Play

Talking to less familiar peers at school can require some planning. Thinking about some topics ahead of time can help you prepare. What is a hobby or interest you have and know a lot about (fashion, sports, music, current events, etc.)? Write it down and include some interesting facts about it. Let the other role-players know what your hobby or interest is so that it can be used in role-play.

Roles

- Three classmates

Role-Play

Imagine you are sitting at a lunch table at school with two other students who are friends with each other. They are liked by other kids in the class and seem easy to get along with. You have never spoken to these kids, and they have not reached out to you.

1. You overhear them talking about this hobby or interest that you have.
2. You listen quietly and look down at your food as you continue to eat.
3. There is a pause in their conversation.
4. You chime in, sharing something about the topic.

Situation 1 (Role-Play Continues):

5. The other kids listen to what you have to say.
6. The kids respond.
7. You continue to make comments, ask questions, and engage in a discussion about the topic.
8. You end the conversation by saying you have to go, and then you say "bye" or wave and leave.

Situation 2 (Role-Play Continues):

5. One of the kids disagrees with what you say.
6. You could stay quiet, but you let them know why you see it a different way.
7. The other kids look at each other, share a signal, get up and walk away.

Reflections

- *What did you think about these two scenes?*
- *Did you like one better than the other? If so, why? If not, why not?*

Cognitive Distortions

If the role-play does not work out as planned and you feel disappointed, think about how you feel and why. Realize that your thoughts can be changed to look at the situation differently.

Personalization

Sometimes people are rude or inconsiderate for reasons that have nothing to do with you, so it is important not to take it personally. For instance, some people will ridicule or brush off someone in front of others to make themselves appear more important. If someone does that to you, it is not because you have done something that deserves ridicule or contempt.

Blaming

You do not need to take responsibility for someone else's poor behavior. It is not your fault that someone else is being unkind or rude.

Scenario 2: Talking to Selected Peers at School

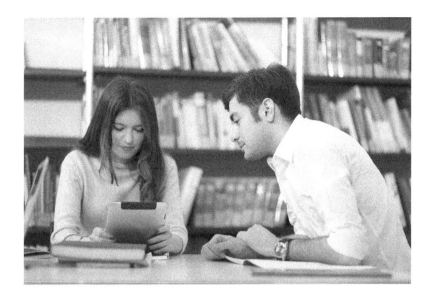

Jesse's Story

"At school a few friendly students say 'hello' and smile at me. One time, I was sitting in a private area upstairs in the school study hall. One of my classmates came to sit with me. He wanted to talk to me, but I kept looking at my computer. I barely responded. He kept using a hand gestures to urge me to say more than the few words I can say when I am in a more secluded area. Then he said, 'You must be studying for that history test.' It was true, but I couldn't engage in conversation."

In Preparation for the Role-Play

Talking to familiar peers at school can require some planning. Thinking about some topics ahead of time can help you prepare. Think about a book you read, a movie you watched, or a social media story you listened to. Write down the name of it and a few details that you remember.

Roles

- Two classmates

Role-Play

In a study room at school, you notice someone else from your grade who is very sociable and curious about others, including you. The student is usually kind and has some good friends. This student has reached out to you in the past, but you did not respond.

1. As you approach the student, you see that she is looking at the same book, movie, or story that you recently read or watched.

2. You sit down across the table from her.
3. You say "Hi" and ask if she's reading or watching anything interesting.

Situation 1 (Role-Play Continues):

4. She says "Hi" and tells you she cannot talk now and gives you a reason.
5. You understand and comment on what she has said.
6. You get back to your own work.

Situation 2 (Role-Play Continues):

4. She answers you.
5. You make a comment or ask another question.
6. She responds, and you both continue to engage in back-and-forth talk with additional questions, answers, and comments.
7. You suggest you both get back to work.
8. She agrees.

Reflections

- *What did you think about these two scenes?*
- *Did you like one better than the other? If so, why? If not, why not?*

Cognitive Distortion

Mind Reading

Do not assume that if someone does not respond the way you want them to that it has anything to do with you. No one can know for sure what people are thinking or why they do what they do. Others can react in a certain way, and we cannot read their minds to know why. You cannot assume people do not like you because they are not able to talk at that time. They may have been preoccupied or studying for an exam.

Jumping to Conclusions

We can easily judge someone with limited information or evidence. You do not always know what makes people react the way they do or what outcome those reactions will lead to. In this particular situation, give the person the benefit of the doubt. She could be a friendly person who is just worried about her test at the moment.

Scenario 3: Being Asked a Question by the Teacher

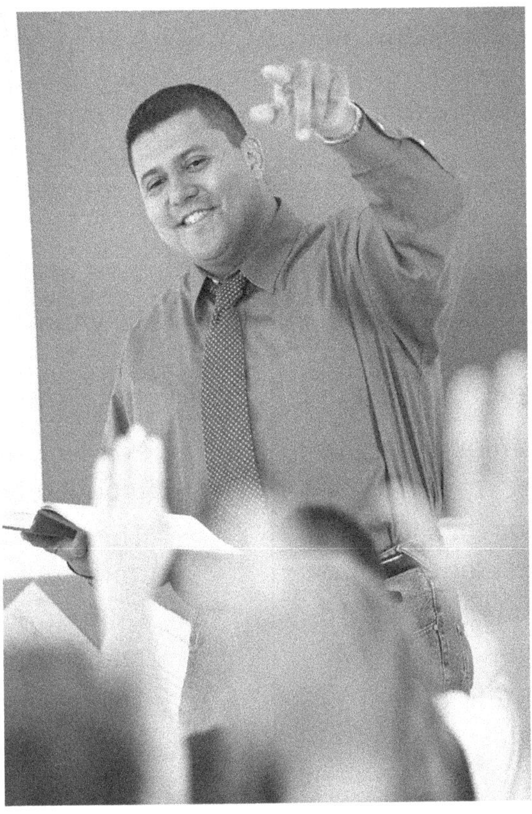

Sandra's Story

"As I continued to withdraw from other students, teachers, and the surroundings at school, I became less preoccupied with getting called on by teachers. However, when a teacher's voice brings me back to reality, I find myself freezing and 'going blank' as I struggle to reply. When I manage to get words out, they are barely audible or comprehensible. One time a teacher called on me and another student gave me the words to say at that moment. Struck with panic, I merely repeated the student's words without processing them while the other students laughed. I ignored their laughs and went back to daydreaming. I wish I had more courage to respond myself."

In Preparation for the Role-Play

Answering a teacher's questions can require some thinking. It helps to know what the teacher will ask ahead of time. In this situation, you need to think about some of your interests and future careers.

Roles

- One teacher
- Three classmates

Role-Play

You are in a class with a teacher who has high expectations. The teacher calls on students but stopped calling on you a few weeks into the class. You never spoke when she did. You wish you could answer at times, but in the past other kids have teased you or said something that hurt your feelings. You know you do the work well independently, but no one else sees it.

1. The teacher has just given an assignment to write what you want to be when you grow up and why.
2. Write down your answer.
3. The teacher calls on you to share your answer while your classmates listen.

Situation 1 (Role-Play Continues):

4. You read your answer aloud to the class.
5. The teacher thanks you for sharing and asks you a question about your choice.
6. You answer her question.
7. The teacher expresses approval of your answer and calls on someone else.

Situation 2 (Role-Play Continues):

4. You look at what you wrote but do not read it aloud.
5. The teacher comes over to your desk and reads your answer for you.
6. Some students sigh, roll their eyes, and whisper to each other.
7. The teacher asks a question.
8. You do not respond verbally but hand the teacher a note with your answer.
9. The teacher had already called on someone else.

Reflections

- *What did you think about these two scenes?*
- *Did you like one better than the other? If so, why? If not, why not?*

Cognitive Distortions

Dichotomous Thinking

Do not think there is only one correct way to answer a question or share an opinion. In this situation, there is no correct answer. You are free to be creative in your response.

Should Statements

Just because you did not answer the question verbally does not mean you failed. Not answering the question does not reflect on your true ability or future performance. When you tell yourself that you should have done something differently, it can prevent you from understanding why you did not. In this situation, the teacher put you on the spot, and you were simply not ready to speak, but you did write your answer.

Scenario 4: Asking the Teacher a Question

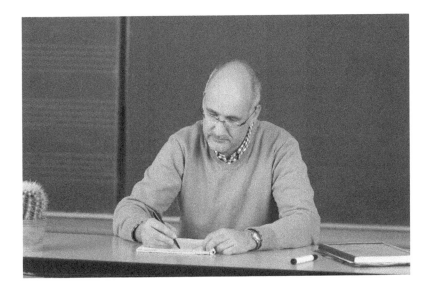

Damien's Story

"While I was taking an exam in English class, my teacher lifted his head and glanced at me. He must have felt I was struggling or thought I hadn't adequately prepared for the exam. After I finished, he came over to my desk to read what I had written. He was intrigued by one of my answers to the fill-in-the-blank section. One of the questions in the section asked us to identify an essential object in the story. I had written the word 'snow.' My teacher told me, in a loud enough voice for others to hear, that my answer to the question shouldn't be 'snow' because snow isn't an object. The student sitting behind me then chuckled. Because I am quiet in class, the teacher struggled to gauge whether I understood the material adequately enough. Also, they know I won't ask questions or disagree with what they say, even if I want to."

In Preparation for the Role-Play

Asking a teacher a question can require some planning. Think about an assignment or project from school that was difficult or confusing. What question would you ask the teacher to help clarify it so you can complete the work?

Roles

- One teacher
- One student

Role-Play

Imagine you are in your classroom and everyone has just been given an assignment to work on independently. The teacher who assigned the activity is assertive and direct with students. You usually keep your head down and try not to get noticed by this teacher.

1. Everyone else in the class begins to work quietly at their desks.
2. You look over the instructions but do not understand one of the steps.
3. You approach the teacher and ask for help.

Situation 1 (Role-Play Continues):

4. Your teacher gives you the answer you need.
5. You ask the teacher a follow-up question.
6. The teacher answers your question and thanks you for asking.
7. You return to your seat to complete your assignment.

Situation 2 (Role-Play Continues):

4. Before you can finish speaking, the teacher cuts you off and tells you not to leave your desk during an in-class assignment.
5. You try asking again.
6. The teacher points to your seat, indicating you should sit down. You return to your desk.
7. You complete the assignment based on your best guess.

Reflections

- *What did you think about these two scenes?*
- *Did you like one better than the other? If so, why? If not, why not?*

Cognitive Distortion

Overgeneralization

If things do not go as you wish, stay open to the possibility things might go differently next time you are in a similar situation. Just because one teacher did not answer your request for information does not mean the next teacher will not.

Personalization

There is no way of knowing why the teacher did not answer. Do not assume that your teacher did not care or that your needs are not important because the teacher did not answer your question. You asked a question and deserved an answer but did not get one. The teacher may have been rushed, feeling ill, or in a bad mood, none of which would have anything to do with you.

Scenario 5: Speaking to Teachers or Staff at School

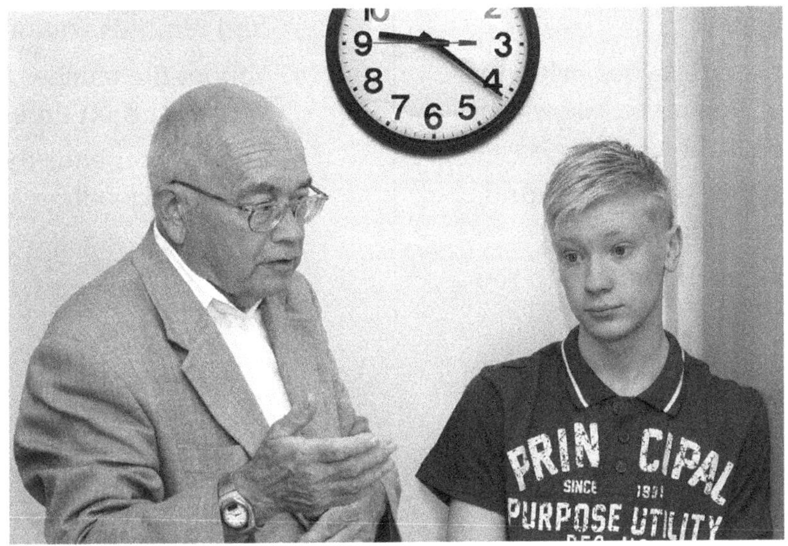

Nick's Story

"On days when math came before homeroom, I had only a few minutes to rush from one end of the school building to the other between those two classes. Since the math classroom was far from homeroom, I was often late to homeroom. The teacher didn't know how far I had to walk, so he handed me a detention slip each time I came late. I would have rather suffered detention than speak to the teacher to defend myself. I didn't want to ask if I could have extra time to travel between classes on the days I had to walk the distance required."

In Preparation for Role-Play

Talking to teachers or staff at school often requires some planning. Think about any time you got in trouble for something (not doing a presentation, coming late, not contributing in a group, etc.). It was not done on purpose.

Roles

- One student
- One teacher

Role-Play

Imagine you have been given a detention slip for something you did at school that you had a good reason for or could not control. In addition, the teacher has requested to meet with you after class.

1. The teacher asks you why this happened.
2. You tell the teacher what happened and explain that it could not be helped.

Situation 1 (Role-Play Continues):

3. The teacher looks at you with understanding.
4. The teacher excuses your behavior this time but warns you she will be stricter in the future.
5. You agree to the compromise and thank her for understanding.
6. The teacher ends the meeting. You both say goodbye.

Situation 2 (Role-Play Continues):

3. The teacher looks at you doubtfully and reminds you of the expectations.
4. You let the teacher know you will try your best next time.
5. The teacher ends the meeting. You both say goodbye.

Reflections

- *What did you think about these two scenes?*
- *Did you like one better than the other? If so, why? If not, why not?*

Cognitive Distortion

Discounting the Positive

Remember that one mistake does not define you or cancel out all other positive experiences. In this scenario, it would be unfortunate to disqualify all the days you did not get in trouble for anything. The circumstances that led to this situation were beyond your control.

Dichotomous Thinking

Situations are not always right or wrong. Sometimes a rule is broken by mistake. When someone believes things are either right or wrong, they are not willing to make exceptions. You cannot control how your teacher sees a situation, but you can choose how you see it, with greater understanding and acceptance.

Scenario 6: Speaking in Groups or in Front of the Class

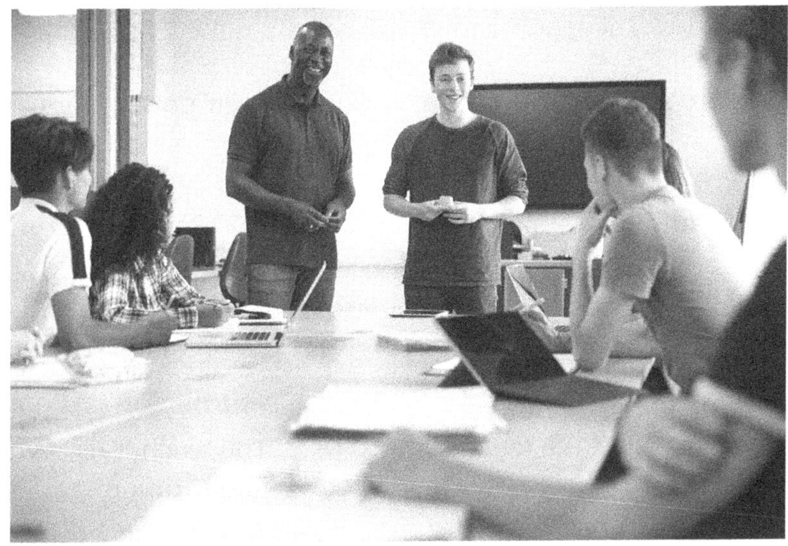

Sam's Story

"I watch other students give presentations in class. It seems easy for them but I describe myself as being 'shut down' during group activities. In one instance, a student in my group said in a negative tone, 'He doesn't speak.' Another student, in agreement with the first student, turned and frowned at me. They both knew I wouldn't defend myself from their hurtful comments and gestures. I worry even more about other students' reactions when I am asked to make a presentation. One of my classes required a presentation from each student. I dreaded this coming event when I would have to speak. Not only did I not prepare for the presentation, but I found it hard to study for exams in the class. I was anxious when I thought about it. I was so concerned that I would have to speak anyway that I ended up going to the teacher's office immediately after class during my free period. I gathered my courage to say, 'It's really hard for me to speak, and I can't present.' Fortunately, he was understanding, and he didn't make me give the presentation and didn't count it toward my grade. I finally opened up to the teacher about having difficulty speaking. It helps when I self-disclose like this."

In Preparation for the Role-Play

Talking in front of class or to a group often requires some planning. Thinking about some topics ahead of time can help you prepare. Think about a topic of your choice. It might be a special item for show-and-tell, a favorite video game or toy, a class project, a vacation, a job you may like when you are older, or any other topic. Write it down and include a few details about it.

Roles

- One teacher
- Two classmates

Role-Play

You are sitting with other students in class getting ready to give your presentation. You have never spoken in front of these kids. The teacher may call on you next.

1. One student asks you what you will talk about in your presentation.
2. You tell him what your topic is.

Situation 1 (Role-Play Continues):

3. The student says something encouraging to you.
4. You ask what they are presenting.
5. You both continue to talk about your topics and how you think the teacher will grade you.
6. The teacher asks you to begin your presentation.
7. You introduce your topic and share the information.

Situation 2 (Role-Play Continues):

3. The student says something unfriendly to you about your topic.
4. You look down at your paper and say you think it is a good topic.
5. The teacher asks you to begin your presentation.
6. You tell the teacher you are not ready.
7. The teacher puts you on the schedule for later in the day.
8. You shake your head OK and want to do well.

Reflections

- *What did you think about these two scenes?*
- *Did you like one better than the other? If so, why? If not, why not?*

Cognitive Distortions

Overgeneralization

Do not let feelings of nervousness keep you from doing something. Just because you may feel uncomfortable at first does not mean that it will always be that way, and presenting to an audience may even turn out not to be as difficult as you initially thought. On the other hand, avoiding something can make a situation worse the next time.

Fortune-Telling/Catastrophizing

Do not predict a negative outcome in the future. What someone says is unrelated to your ability to perform or cope with the stress of a challenge. Although something feels difficult, if you try and see a different outcome, you could be happy.

Scenario 7: Talking to Family Members at Home When Others Are Present

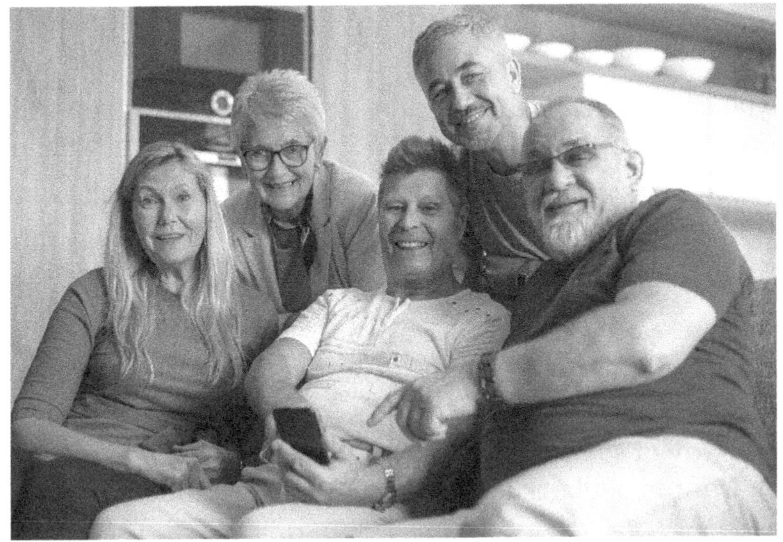

Amanda's Story

"My mother has a group of friends who visit our home once a week. She likes to show pictures of the family and this time they were asking about me. I usually stay in my bedroom with the door slightly open if I want to get my mom's attention when she comes upstairs. She allows me to remain silent and ignore visitors. Sometimes I can't get her attention without speaking loud enough for her to hear me when she is with the group. So I don't say anything. My fear is that my mother's friends would want me to come out of my room and greet them and then I would have to respond."

In Preparation for the Role-Play

Talking to people who visit your house may require some planning about what to say. What is something going on at school, at home, or in your personal life right now that is exciting, interesting, or disturbing to you? It could be an event involving you or someone else that you are paying attention to, like a challenging assignment, a school dance, an athletic event, a new friend, or something else.

Roles

- One child/teen
- One family friend

Role-Play

You were studying in your room all day, and just as you were thinking it might be nice to have a snack from the kitchen, you hear the voices of your parents' friends entering your home. You are hungry, and you will pass by the guests and your parents on the way to the kitchen.

1. You walk to the kitchen avoiding eye contact.
2. One of the guests expresses excitement over seeing you.

Situation 1 (Role-Play Continues):

3. They insist you sit down with them.
4. You sit down.
5. One of the guests asks how you are doing.
6. You shrug and look away.
7. The guest pressures you to say something about what is going on in your life.
8. You move in a way or say something to signal you want to get back to studying.
9. The guest expresses their disappointment that you are busy and unavailable to give them an update.
10. You get up and leave.

Situation 2 (Role-Play Continues):

3. They ask if you will sit down with them and say hello.
4. You approach them and sit or stand.
5. The guest asks what's new.
6. You share something that is going on in your life.
7. They ask a question or share a story that relates to what you said.
8. You ask a follow-up question or make a comment.
9. They respond.
10. You tell them you have to go and say goodbye.

Cognitive Distortion

Magnification/Minimization

Sometimes conversations are uncomfortable, but that does not mean you have done something wrong. Even if you walk away with a negative feeling, you can still appreciate how brave it was to participate and express your needs.

What If?

We cannot predict what people will ask us or what they will want to talk about in a conversation. What if you are not sure what to say? It is OK to let the person know. This is a common situation for many people. No one knows everything all the time. You can say, "I don't know" or "I'm not sure."

Scenario 8: Talking to Family Members While in Unfamiliar Places

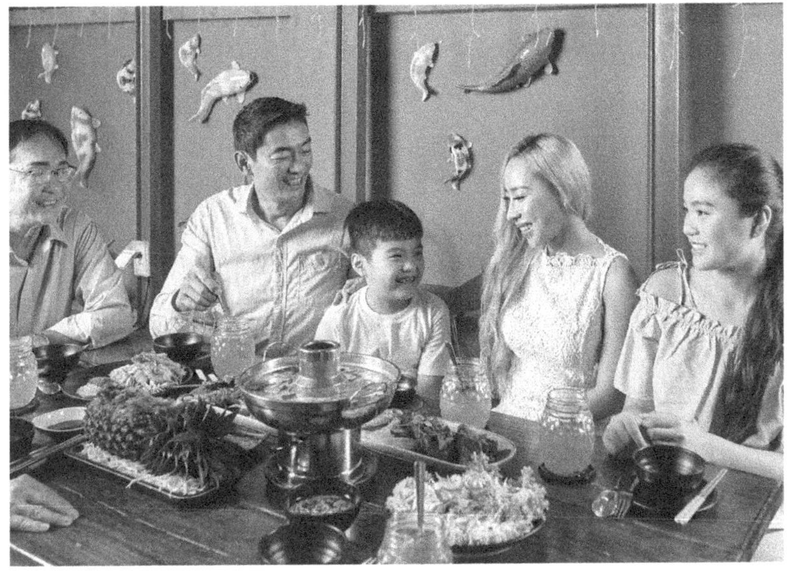

Abby's Story

"At restaurants, I only feel comfortable speaking to family members from the table if no one is within hearing distance. I am self-conscious most of the time, imagining gazes on me at restaurants. I remember when my family and I were out for dinner together after my middle school graduation. If anyone unfamiliar was nearby, I wouldn't speak to my family. At the restaurant, a group of classmates recognized me and shouted praise for my receiving an academic award. I didn't acknowledge these classmates and sat at the table with my family in silence. I didn't want the classmates to hear me talk. It was difficult to change my image as the girl who doesn't talk."

In Preparation for the Role-Play

Talking to family members in unfamiliar places when others are nearby may require some planning. What is something you are good at that you might receive praise for? You could choose an art project, sports, a math test, or anything else.

Roles

- Two classmates
- One family member

Role-Play

Imagine that you have just won an award for this at a school assembly and your family has taken you out to a restaurant to celebrate. You are proud of your work. You see one of your classmates enter the restaurant. This classmate is not someone you talk to at school, but the classmate is always kind to you and seen as a generous and caring person by everyone.

1. Your classmate sees you and smiles.

Situation 1 (Role-Play Continues):

2. You sit back in your seat.
3. The classmate approaches and congratulates you on your award.
4. You look down at your food.
5. Your classmate leaves, and you relax a little. You do not talk for the rest of the meal now that you think you might be overheard.

Situation 2 (Role-Play Continues):

2. You smile back.
3. The classmate approaches and congratulates you on getting an award in school and asks you what it was for.
4. You thank your classmate and tell them about the award. You also introduce the classmate to your family.
5. One family member responds.
6. The classmate says it was nice to meet everyone and then goes back to their family.
7. You say "bye."

Reflections

- *What did you think about these two scenes?*
- *Did you like one better than the other? If so, why? If not, why not?*

Cognitive Distortion

Discounting the Positive

Uncomfortable situations may sometimes make you explain away your successes and positive experiences. Another option is to embrace your accomplishments and the rewards they bring from others.

Emotional Reasoning

If you are known as the kid who does not talk in school, you may feel embarrassed if a student hears you speak and try to avoid it. Do not let your attitudes or judgments dictate your actions and prevent you from talking to your family outside the home.

Scenario 9: Talking to Family Members Who Do Not Live With Me (e.g., grandparent, cousin)

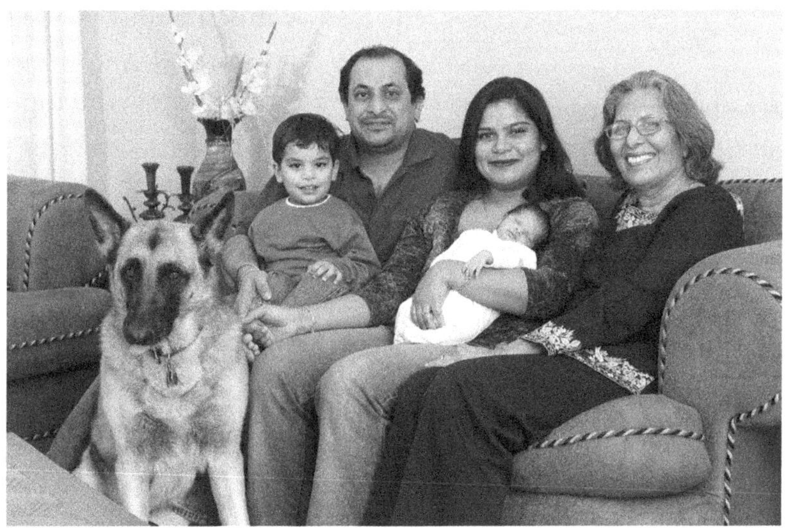

Lily's Story

"At extended family visits, usually during holidays, I barely greet my aunts and uncles upon entering their house. When my aunts and uncles try to engage me in conversation, I don't join in. I am so self-conscious that I am not going to say the right thing or that I will "mess up" that I can hardly respond. They must think I am rude or intimidated. I speak to my cousins when I visit them but only while we are in a room with the door closed and the adults are in a different place. I feel that I would be interrogated and judged by them, and I am afraid of what people may think of me. I feel like they're smarter than me and they know more than I do. I think I wouldn't be able to add anything to the conversation and would sound silly. I find it difficult to know what to say and what not to say."

In Preparation for the Role-Play

Talking to less familiar family members can require some planning. Thinking about some topics ahead of time can help you prepare. What are some topics that you know a lot about? Share this with the other role-players to use in the activity.

Roles

- One child/teen
- Two family members

Role-Play

You are visiting some family members, and you go off on your own to a private area where you will not be disturbed. After a while, one of your parents calls your name from where they are sitting with other family members. You approach the group.

Situation 1:

1. A family member asks you a question about a topic that you know a lot about.
2. You answer.
3. They are interested in what you are saying and ask another question.
4. You engage in back-and-forth talk with additional questions, answers, and comments.
5. They thank you for sharing the information.
6. You say thank you and go back to what you were doing.

Situation 2:

1. A family member asks you a question about a topic that you do not know much about.
2. You think about something to say but don't know the topic.
3. Before you can say that you don't know much about the topic, someone else chimes in with an answer about the topic.
4. Others nod in approval.
5. You tell them you have to go and say goodbye.

Reflections

- *What did you think about these two scenes?*
- *Did you like one better than the other? If so, why? If not, why not?*

Cognitive Distortions

Emotional Reasoning

If you are nervous about a conversation, that is not a sign that the conversation will go badly or that you will mess up. You may be reacting emotionally to assumptions you made about the people you're speaking with instead of who they really are. In this situation, you may have felt you were being judged, but it is possible someone was just chiming in or sharing their ideas.

Unfair Comparisons

People are knowledgeable about something because they either are regularly involved in it or are interested in it. It is unfair to judge yourself based on someone else's measure of knowledge because you cannot know what goes into their learning. It works the other way too; other people do not know at first glance how hard you work at something or the time you take to learn it.

Scenario 10: Talking on the Phone to Parents and/or Siblings

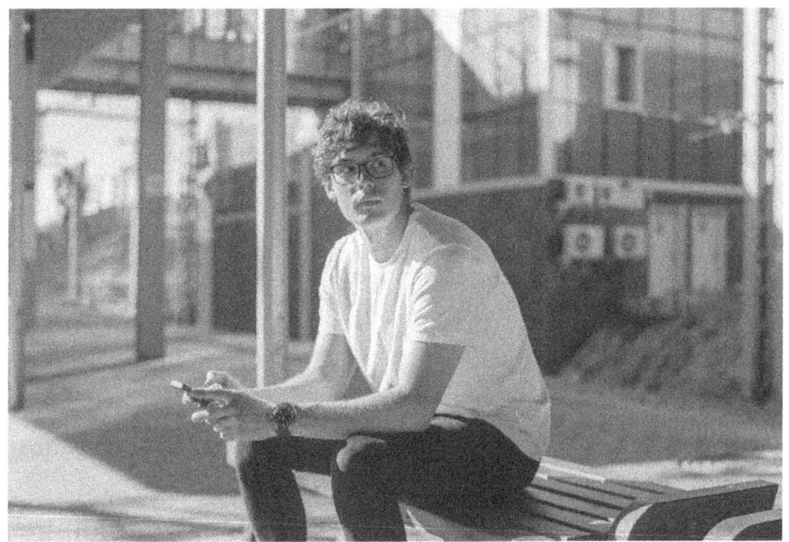

Ken's Story

"I avoid talking on the phone to my parents and brother in the presence of others. I don't answer my mobile phone, even if it is them, while in public. A simple call would provoke anxiety and make me feel exposed to other people judging my voice and manner of speech. While at a bus stop, I answered my phone without realizing how anxious I would become when speaking in front of others. I remember whispering into the receiver and the person on the other line couldn't hear me and asked me to repeat myself. When I tried to raise my voice above the street noise, I struggled to talk as I strained to get the words out, and I panicked about how I sounded to others. I cared too much about what others thought."

In Preparation for the Role-Play

Talking to family members on the phone when others are around may be challenging if you do not want others to hear what you are saying. You can try to distance yourself or speak in a quieter voice. Think of reasons that your family would call you. Write a phone conversation you had or that you could imagine having with someone in your family.

Roles

- Two strangers
- One family member

Role-Play

You are sitting at a public place next to someone who is reading a book. Your phone rings.

1. You take out your phone.
2. The person reading the book glances at your phone and then looks back at their book.
3. You see it is your family member calling.

Situation 1 (Role-Play Continues):

4. You answer the phone.
5. The person reading the book glances at you, frowns disapprovingly and then looks down at their book.
6. Your family member tells you why they are calling.
7. You respond to the family member.
8. The person next to you sighs audibly and shifts their body away from you.
9. You tell the family member that you cannot talk now. The family member ends the call.

Situation 2 (Role-Play Continues):

4. You answer the phone.
5. Your family member tells you why they are calling.
6. You respond to the family member on the phone and continue your conversation in a quiet voice.
7. The person next to you looks up at you for a moment and then returns to their book.
8. You let your family member know when you will be home, and then you end the call.

Reflections

- *What did you think about these two scenes?*
- *Did you like one better than the other? If so, why? If not, why not?*

Cognitive Distortion

Mind Reading

It is impossible to know what someone else might be thinking. A glance from a stranger could indicate an emotional response they are having to something you are saying or doing. It could also be a response to something that has nothing to do with you. It is also important to consider how much to invest in other people's judgments of you. This may not be worth your time or energy.

Jumping to Conclusions

Speaking on the phone when others are nearby might feel uncomfortable. Do not assume that others listening in will judge you. They may simply mind their own business and pay no attention. They may be focused on what they are doing or thinking so that you can focus on your conversation in peace.

Scenario 11: Speaking With Familiar Family Friends

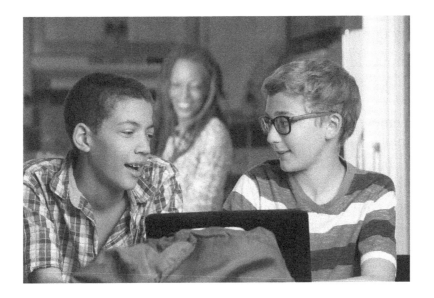

Ryan's Story

"From time to time, I visit close family friends of my parents. They live in another state, so that's why I don't see them too often. My mother's friend is nice, and she has a son who is 2 years younger than me and also kind. I feel more comfortable with him than other kids because we are somewhat similar. I can relate to him. I speak with him and his mother, making basic comments and greetings. I feel less pressure to speak and end up acting more freely around them. I think this may be due to feelings of being appreciated as a friend and not feeling that I am being analyzed or judged. This is rarely the case."

In Preparation for the Role-Play

Talking to familiar friends of the family can be enjoyable. What is an activity that you like to do with your friends that a grown-up would have to take you to or go with you? What is an activity that you do not like doing but other friends and family like doing?

Roles

- Two friends
- One family member

Role-Play

You arrive at your friend's house, and their family is getting ready to go out for the day with you. Your friend told you it would be a surprise, and you are hoping it is something you like doing.

1. Your friend's family member says, "Guess what we're doing today!" to you and your friend.

Situation 1 (Role-Play Continues):

2. Your friend immediately, enthusiastically shouts out something you like to do.
3. His family member asks you if you want to do that.
4. You say that you do like that and want to do it.
5. There is a short conversation about the activity. You may add comments, share stories, and ask questions.
6. A family member suggests getting ready to go. You agree.

Situation 2 (Role-Play Continues):

2. Your friend immediately, enthusiastically shouts out the option that you do not like.
3. Your friends' family member asks if you want to do that.
4. You really do not want to go to that place, so you offer another idea.
5. Your friend's family member tells you it is already paid for so you have to go there this time.
6. You understand and say OK.
7. Your friend reassures you that it will be fun.
8. A family member suggests getting ready to go. You agree.

Reflections

- *What did you think about these two scenes?*
- *Did you like one better than the other? If so, why? If not, why not?*

Cognitive Distortion

Fortune-Telling

Having to do something or go someplace that you did not like in the past can be upsetting or scary. You may worry that you will not have a good time again. Expecting to have a bad time can prevent you from having a good time and enjoying yourself.

Discounting the Positive

There are usually positive and negative parts to a situation. Just because you do not like the place where you are going, that does not mean you cannot have a good time. You like your friend and spending time with them and your family. Do not make a negative situation diminish a positive one.

Scenario 12: Speaking to at Least One Babysitter or Caregiver (not family member)

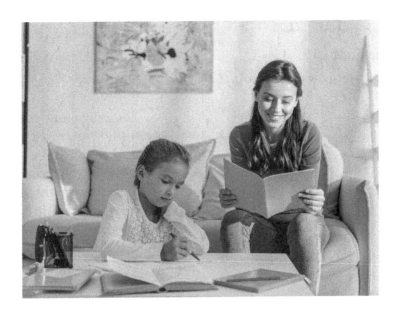

Jasmin's Story

"Before I turned 12, I had a babysitter. I spent time playing and interacting with my babysitter, even without speaking. During that period, there was less pressure at home to speak using more complex thoughts. Those who entered the house understood me as a quiet but active child. When I started thinking that I was expected to speak to the babysitter, I shut down and even stopped playing. I probably missed out on having some fun after I changed my behavior toward the babysitter."

In Preparation for the Role-Play

Talking to someone who is watching you or taking care of you can be fun if you are more familiar with them. If it is someone who you do not know as well, you may need to do some planning to get ready. When you are stuck at home, what are some things you like to do alone or with someone else: watch a movie, play a game, write, learn something new, etc.?

Roles

- One child/teen
- One babysitter/caregiver

Role-Play

Your parents are getting ready to leave and to your surprise, a new babysitter has just arrived.

1. The babysitter/caregiver says hello and introduces themself.

Situation 1 (Role-Play Continues):

2. You greet the babysitter/caregiver.
3. The babysitter/caregiver asks about your school and hobbies.
4. You answer the questions.
5. The babysitter/caregiver asks if you want to play a game or watch a movie together.
6. You tell the babysitter/caregiver what you would like to do but that you are busy with something else and will try to play later.
7. The babysitter/caregiver says OK, and you go to your room to finish what you were doing.

Situation 2 (Role-Play Continues):

2. You do not respond.
3. The babysitter/caregiver asks again, waiting for a response.
4. You look away and after a minute of deciding if you'll answer, you say your name.
5. The babysitter/caregiver smiles and thinks you must be busy. They tell you that they will be at your house for a while and to come back if you want to play something or watch TV. You wave and smile back and then leave to go to your room.

Cognitive Distortion

Should Statements

If you tell yourself you should act in a certain way or do certain things but do not want to, that can cause conflict. You are not obliged to do things that make you feel uncomfortable, but pushing yourself to engage in new experiences that are safe may provide enjoyment. Using "should" or "should not" statements can cause you to miss out on potentially positive experiences or relationships.

Unfair Comparisons

At times you will be put in new situations with less familiar people and may worry about being compared to others. You may wonder what to say and how to say it, and if the new people will like you. Remember, each person brings their own experiences and value to a situation. People usually take time to get to know each other before becoming friends. You are unique and have your own qualities to share.

Scenario 13: Speaking With Other Kids Whom I Do Not Know

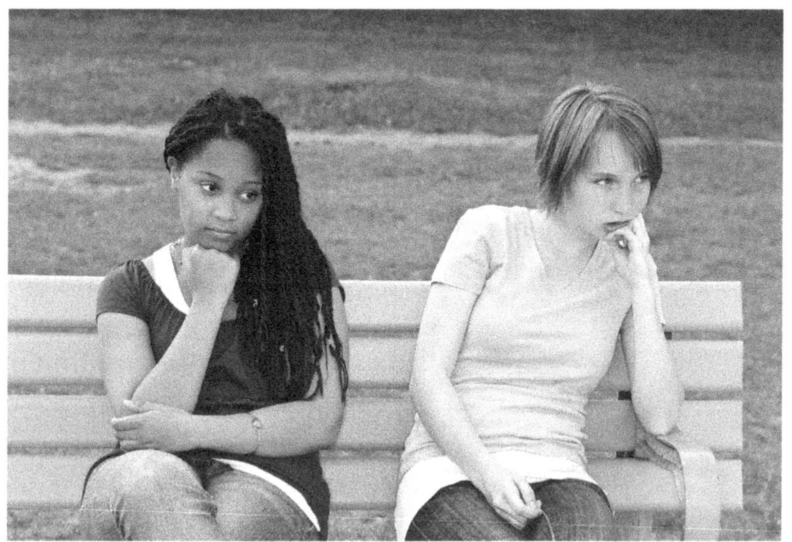

Lena's Story

"I hang out with a small group of neighborhood friends who don't attend my high school and are a year younger than me. Sometimes one of my friends brings someone around whom I don't know. One time a new kid came to my neighborhood to meet their friend and I was there. When my friend had to go home I was left alone with the new kid. She looked at me, wanting to talk, but I looked away. She thought I wasn't friendly. New people often think I am unfriendly by my quiet behavior. It would be good to branch out and make new friends if I felt more confident about talking."

In Preparation for the Role-Play

Talking to other kids you do not know can be stressful. Think about a friend you have and the first time you met that friend. Remember that at one time you did not know that person either. Think about some questions you could ask to get to know someone better.

Roles

- Three peers

Role-Play

You have gone to visit your friend, and to your surprise, they have another guest over. Your friend introduces the two of you, and then is unexpectedly called away by a family member, leaving you and the other guest alone.

1. The guest looks at you and smiles.
2. There is silence.

Situation 1 (Role-Play Continues):

3. You ask a question about how this guest and your friend know each other.
4. The guest responds and asks you the same question.
5. The conversation continues until your friend comes back and then you tell your friend what you were talking about.

Situation 2 (Role-Play Continues):

3. The guest asks you if you know where the friend went and why they left.
4. You look in the direction your friend left but do not answer.
5. The guest asks why you are not answering.
6. You tell the guest you do not know and that the friend did not tell you.
7. Your friend walks in, and you say "now we can find out."

Reflections

- *What did you think about these two scenes?*
- *Did you like one better than the other? If so, why? If not, why not?*

Cognitive Distortion

Blaming

When there is an expectation to have a conversation, the responsibility is not all on you. You may or may not choose to initiate or respond. The other person might feel uncomfortable in the situation themself and stay quiet. People usually try their best with what they can do at the time. If something is beyond your comfort level, do not blame yourself or anyone else. Instead, work on improving the skills.

Selective Abstraction

Being overly focused on one thing can make it harder to do something else. Thinking about how you are going to get the words out or talk to someone new can limit your ability to think about the situation and say your thoughts. Worrying about how others will react to what you say can derail the interaction.

Scenario 14: Speaking With Family Friends Whom I Do Not Know

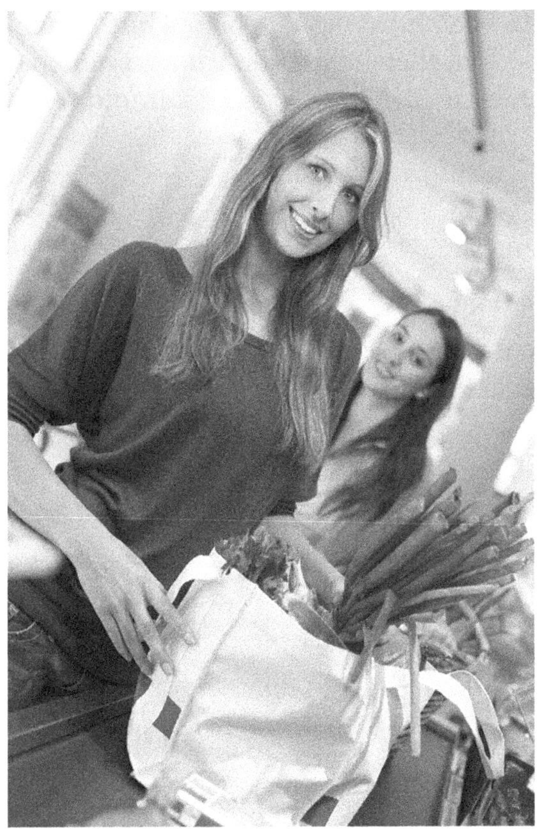

Jane's Story

"Anytime I go to the supermarket and see a neighbor or family friend there, I stay quiet. If I notice them, I just look away at something on the shelf in the store, even if I am comfortable and content before then. If I am with a family member, I stand behind them and let them do the talking. One time when I was alone in the store, a neighbor approached me and I froze because I wasn't sure what to say. She asked me if something was wrong or if I didn't like her. She left me alone. In those moments, I would find something else to distract me and avoid saying hello."

In Preparation for the Role-Play

Talking to people you do not know can be challenging. Write down some simple phrases you can use for a casual, short conversation. It may be a greeting, questions about how someone is doing, comments about the weather or your immediate surroundings, mentioning a sporting event or something in popular culture, or anything else that does not invite deep conversation.

Roles

- One child/teen
- One acquaintance

Role-Play

You are in line at the supermarket when an acquaintance of your parents takes the place behind you. This is someone you have been introduced to before but you do not know well. The few times you have encountered this person, they have been very animated and vocally expressive. If you have a conversation with someone like that, you think it might draw attention to you.

1. The person greets you, using your name.

Situation 1 (Role-Play Continues):

2. You look down at the floor.
3. They make a comment about your silence and ask if you are okay.
4. You look up and nod your head up and down to indicate yes.
5. The person says, that's good, and then they ask you to say hello to your parents when you see them.
6. After you check out you wave goodbye.

Situation 2 (Role-Play Continues):

2. You greet the person.
3. They ask you a question or make a comment.
4. You respond and add a comment or question of your own.
5. They respond.
6. They ask you to say hello to your parents when you see them.
7. You agree.
8. You both stand quietly until it is your turn to check out.
9. After you check out you say goodbye.

Reflections

- *What did you think about these two scenes?*
- *Did you like one better than the other? If so, why? If not, why not?*

Cognitive Distortion

What If?

Sometimes you may not know what to say to someone whom you do not know well. You may be concerned that the person who is trying to talk with you may judge what you say or how you say it. Instead of wondering what if you make a mistake or say something wrong, not saying anything at all can call more attention to you than responding with a simple acknowledgment.

Labeling

Putting a negative label on yourself can make you afraid to speak up. Each person has both positive and negative traits. Do not let labels affect you. What you think of yourself is what matters. Thinking positively about yourself is always best.

Scenario 15: Speaking With My Doctor or Dentist

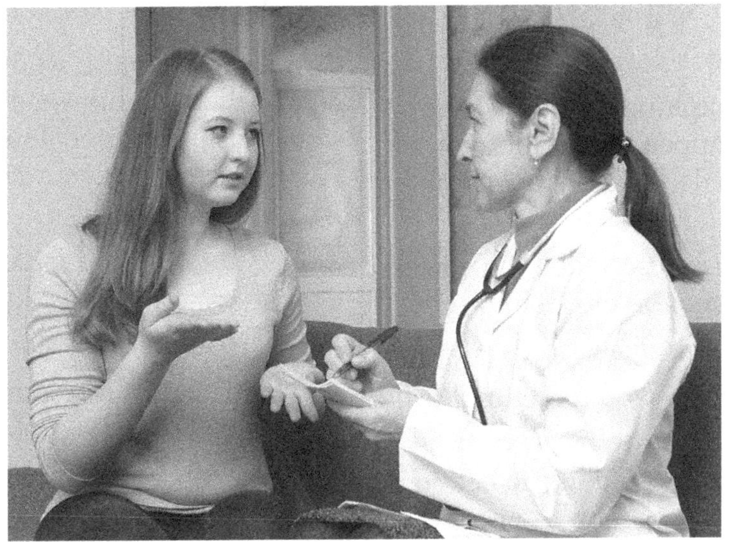

Kayla's Story

"When I was a kid, going to the doctor or dentist was uncomfortable but not as bad as it could have been because my parents went with me, and my mother usually did all the talking. Being quiet didn't matter in that scenario. Now that I am older and need to express my thoughts about treatment, I have trouble. One time at the physical therapist's office, I didn't speak up to ask for help when I didn't know how to do a certain exercise. That gave the impression that I didn't care when I actually did care. Not speaking is often misinterpreted as not caring. I'm just not comfortable asking for help when I need it."

In Preparation for the Role-Play

Talking to professionals for treatment requires that you let them know what you need. Have you ever been hurt or gotten sick in a way that affected your participation in an activity you enjoy, like a sport, dance, gaming, or a social activity? Think of a time you went to your doctor and needed to explain what was happening to you.

Roles

- One child/teen
- One parent
- One doctor

Role-Play

You have an injury or are ill and are at the doctor's office with your parent. Because of your injury, you are unable to participate in the activity of your choice and think you may never get better again.

1. The doctor asks you what is wrong in front of your parent.

Situation 1 (Role-Play Continues):

2. You look at your parent.
3. Your parent explains what is wrong and how it happened and that you are unable to do the activity of your choice.
4. Your parent asks you to tell the doctor how much pain you are feeling.
5. You respond with a few words.
6. The doctor thanks you for letting them know.
7. Your parent says you'd like to get back to your activities as soon as possible.
8. The doctor says they will see what you can do.
9. You say thank you and wave goodbye as you leave with your parent.

Situation 2 (Role-Play Continues):

2. You explain what is wrong and how it happened. You add that it is preventing you from doing the activity of your choice.
3. The doctor tells you they share that interest and makes a comment.
4. You respond with a question, comment, or story.
5. The doctor responds and says they will see what you can do to get back to it as soon as possible.
6. You say thank you and wave goodbye as you leave with your parent.

Reflections

- *What did you think about these two scenes?*
- *Did you like one better than the other? If so, why? If not, why not?*

Cognitive Distortion

Overgeneralization

It may be that the adults in the room, especially where parents are present, often lead discussions on your behalf. But that is not how it always has to be. It is worthy to speak up for yourself so that doctors and others know how to help you. Do not assume that you will always have to rely on those who care for you to express your needs.

Fortune-Telling/Catastrophizing

It is possible you have had trouble expressing yourself to a doctor in the past. However, that does not mean it will always be that way. In this situation, if you make your needs known, the doctor will understand you. You might think of important details that your parent did not.

Scenario 16: Speaking to Store Clerks or Waiters

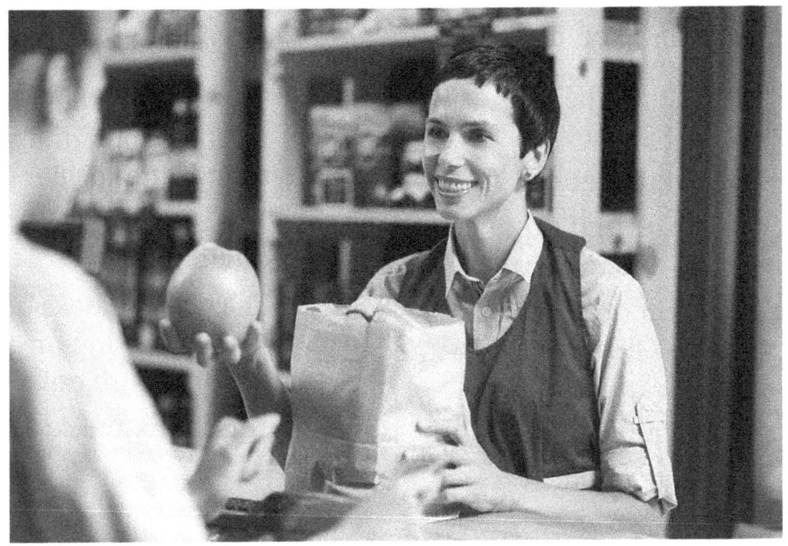

Brittney's Story

"When I was younger, my limited verbal communication did not stop me from getting the food I wanted because my father ordered food for the table at restaurants. At stores, I didn't speak to store clerks. Now being a teen, I remember a recent time when I needed to return something and my parents weren't there. I didn't feel comfortable telling the store clerk why I wanted to return the item, so I didn't speak up for myself. Instead of returning it, I took it back home."

In Preparation for the Role-Play

Talking to store clerks or waiters can be difficult but helps you get what you want. What is an item that you would like to have that you could save up money to purchase? It could be clothing, a game, a collector's item, or anything.

Roles

- One customer
- One cashier

Role-Play

After saving up money for months, you are finally able to take your cash to the store and make your purchase. You approach the cashier with the item.

1. The cashier seems distracted and looks at their watch, sighs, and tells you how much you owe.
2. You hand the cashier your money.

3. The cashier gives you change and the receipt, but the amount is less than what it should be. The cashier owes you an extra dollar.

Situation 1 (Role-Play Continues):

4. You tell the cashier that the change is not correct.
5. The cashier looks at the receipt.
6. The cashier apologizes and explains that they have had a long day.
7. You make a comment and reassure the cashier that it is OK.
8. The cashier gives you the correct amount that goes with your receipt.
9. You thank the cashier and leave

Situation 2 (Role-Play Continues):

4. You point to the amount due to you on the receipt and show how much money the cashier gave you.
5. The cashier looks at you and sighs audibly.
6. The cashier looks at the receipt without saying anything and gives you the extra dollar owed to you.
7. You thank the cashier and leave.

Reflections

- *What did you think about these two scenes?*
- *Did you like one better than the other? If so, why? If not, why not?*

Cognitive Distortion

Personalization

There are many reasons why people act the way they do, most of which have nothing to do with you. If someone seems upset, that might be for a specific reason that has nothing to do with you. It might also be because they are just rude. In that case, do not take it personally. Finish what you need to do and do not let what someone else says or does bother you.

Should Statements

People who are serving the public, such as clerks or waiters, are often thought to do their job correctly. However, anyone can make a mistake. Thinking that you should be quiet when someone makes a mistake that affects you is a problem. You should speak up to protect yourself or make your needs known.

Scenario 17: Talking When in Clubs, Teams, or Organized Activities Outside of School

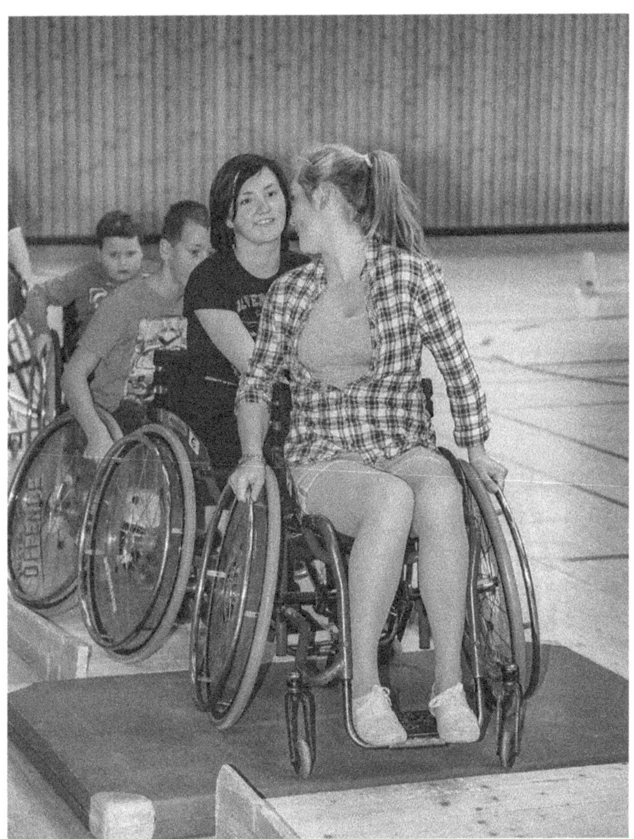

Chris' Story

"My parents enrolled me in a basketball program at the community center. I didn't engage with the other players and distanced myself from connecting with them due to my fear of being judged. During practice, I felt self-conscious and gave it little effort. After the program manager complained about my lack of participation, I wanted to quit. I convinced my parents to take me out with the promise that I would play one-on-one basketball with my father. I was honest with them about my anxiety and difficulty speaking."

In Preparation for the Role-Play

Talking to others during clubs, teams, or organized activities outside of school can present challenges. You want to fit in and have friends. If you were to join any club outside of school, what would it be? Why does it interest you? How would it challenge you? Think about these questions to prepare for conversation.

Roles

- Two peers

Role-Play

You are in a club outside of school and everyone is engaged in the activity. You are next to someone performing the same activity. Conversation is welcome but not necessary.

Situation 1:

1. You notice them performing a task with a skill you do not have but wish you did.
2. You decide to take the lead and initiate with a comment on the person's skills.
3. The peer says thank you and asks you if you want to learn how they do that.
4. You say yes and give it a try. The peer seems to like coaching you. This person may become a new friend.

Situation 2:

1. The peer turns to you at the club and asks if you want to join in an activity.
2. You are new to the club and say yes by nodding your head.
3. The peer asks you a question about yourself.
4. You could stay quiet, but you decide to answer and then ask the peer the same question.
5. You let this peer know that talking is not easy for you sometimes.
6. The peer thanks you for saying that and says it is that way for them too at times. You continue with the activity.
7. You both talk a little longer and then it is time to go.
8. You say goodbye after the activity and hope to see each other next time.

Reflections

- *What did you think about these two scenes?*
- *Did you like one better than the other? If so, why? If not, why not?*

Cognitive Distortion

Unfair Comparisons

If someone has a skill that you do not have, it does not mean they are better than you. It might mean they have something they can teach you. Being preoccupied with who is better than whom can get in the way of improving or helping others to improve. Connecting with someone else who has similar interests as you can be the start of a friendship.

Dichotomous Thinking

Sometimes you may think experiences can be either positive or negative. If you are meeting someone new, you may worry that it will be a good experience or a bad one. In reality, things are usually not one way or another, but a combination. Take a chance knowing that you can always learn from experiences that do not initially go as planned.

Photo Cards

Photo cards can be used to choose and assume a new identity for any role-play. Cut (and possibly laminate) and tape/place near the individual to assume the new role of the person in the photo.

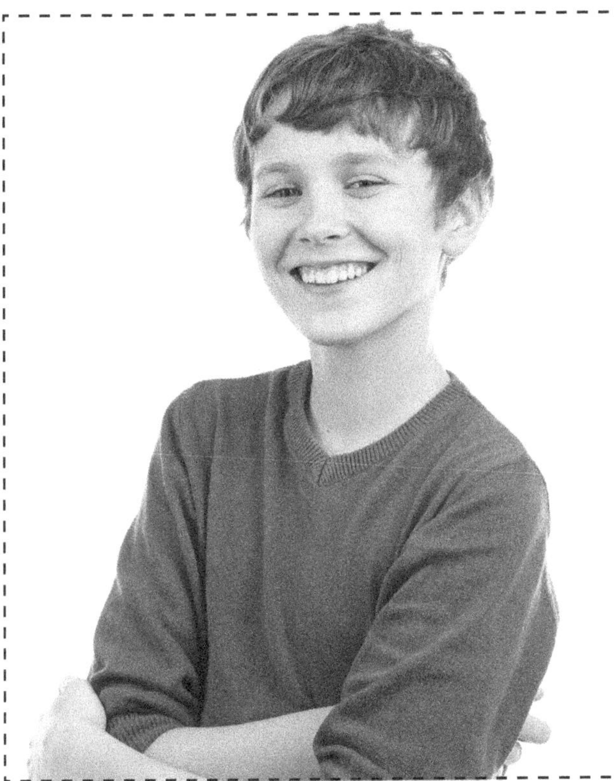

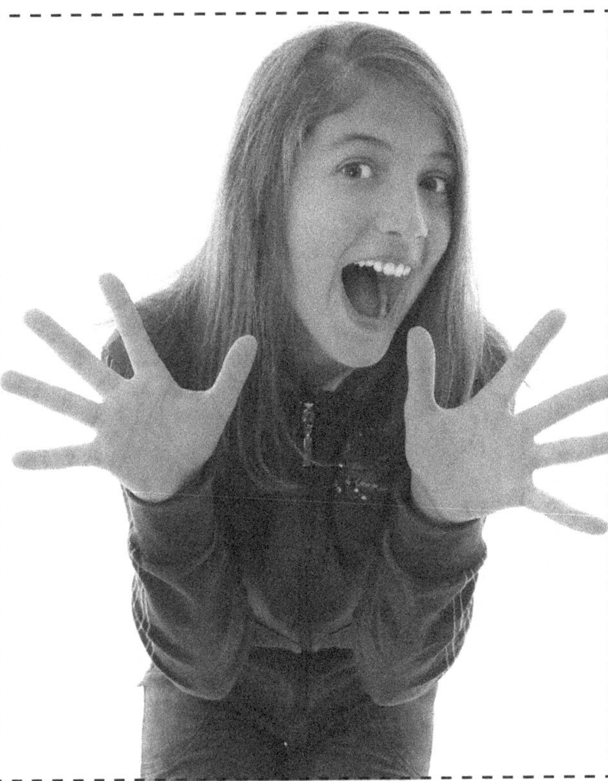

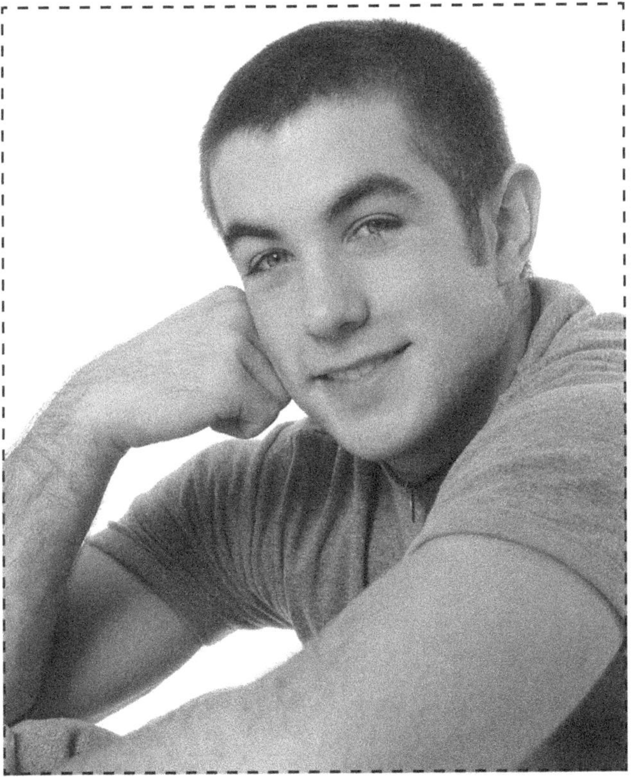

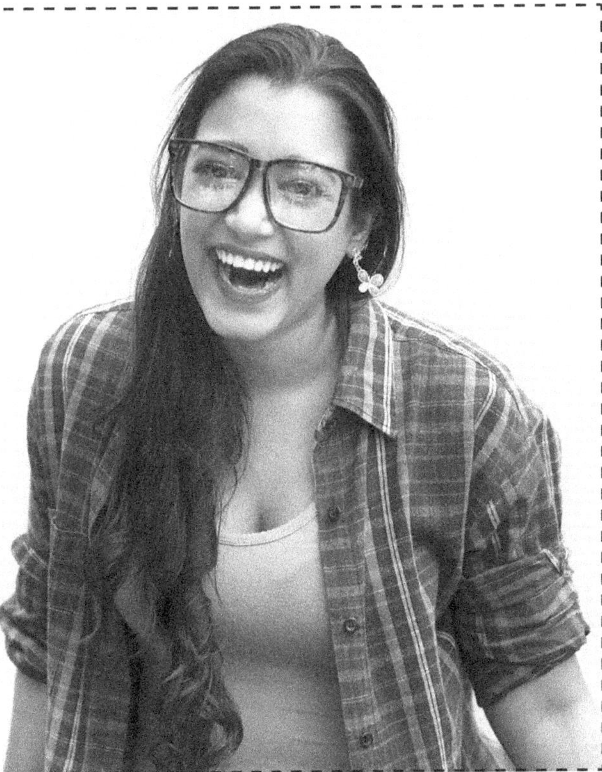

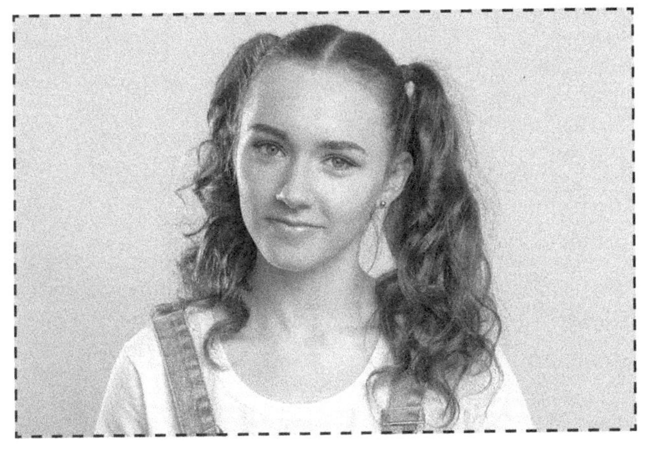
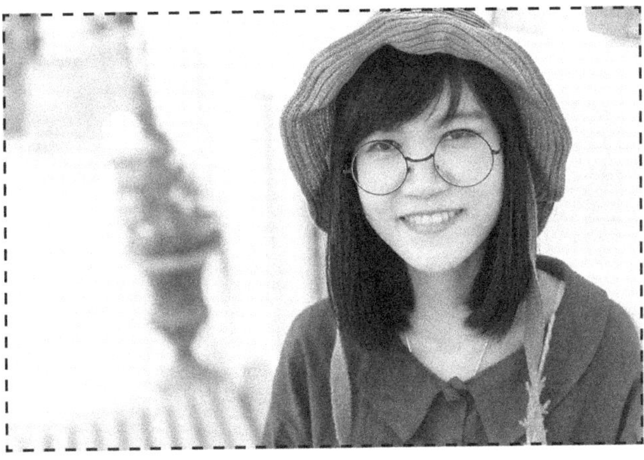
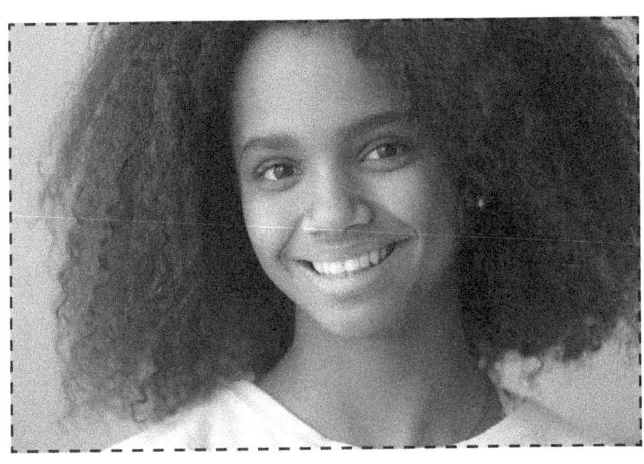
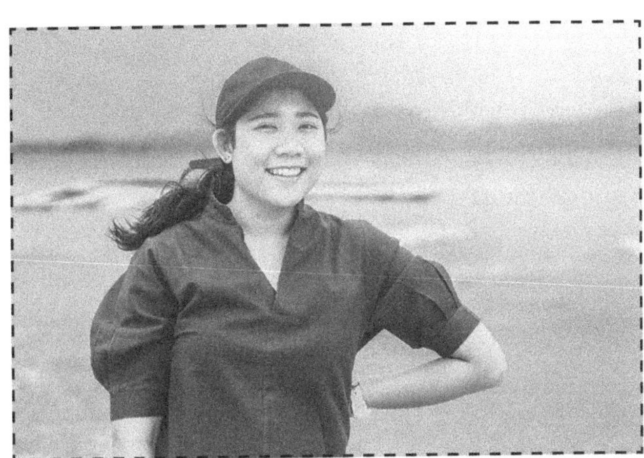
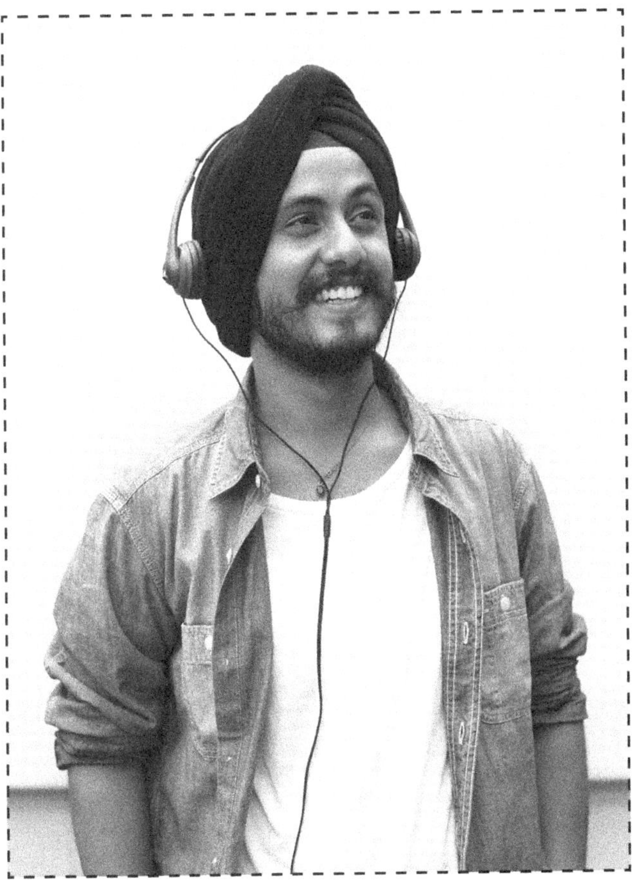
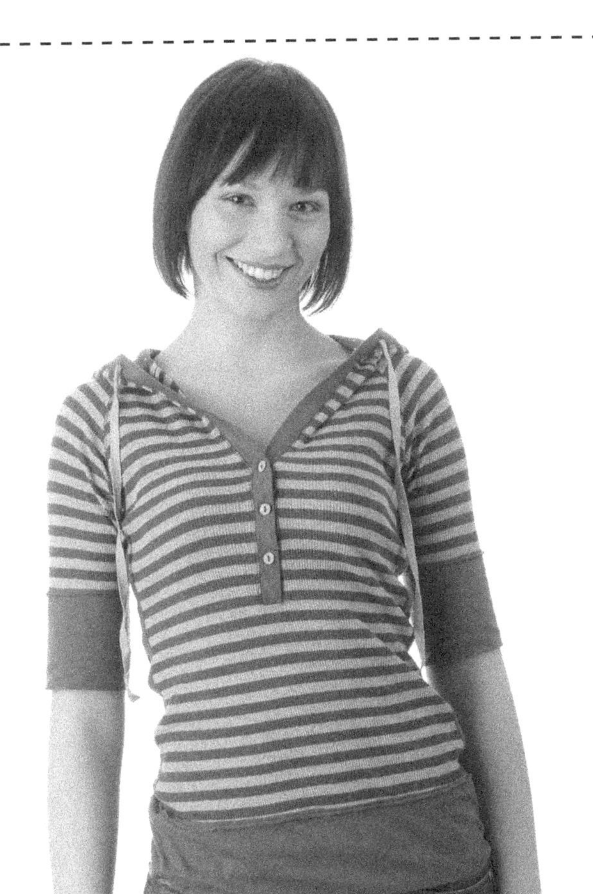

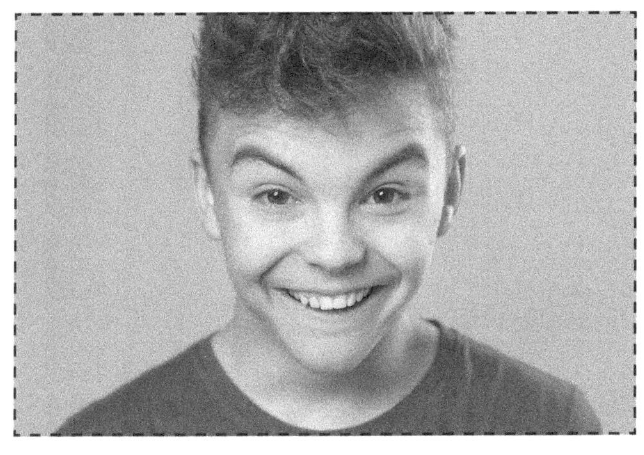
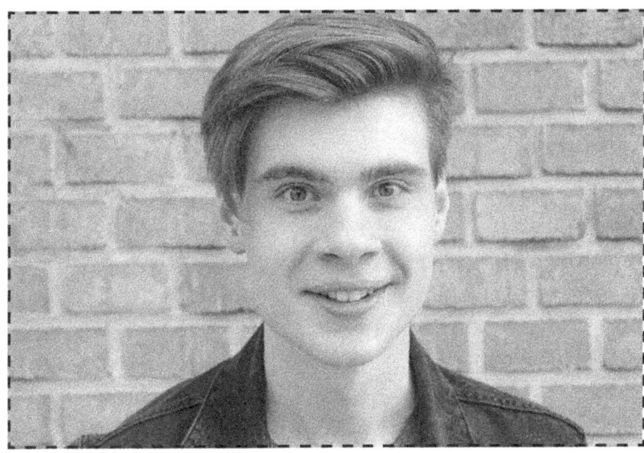
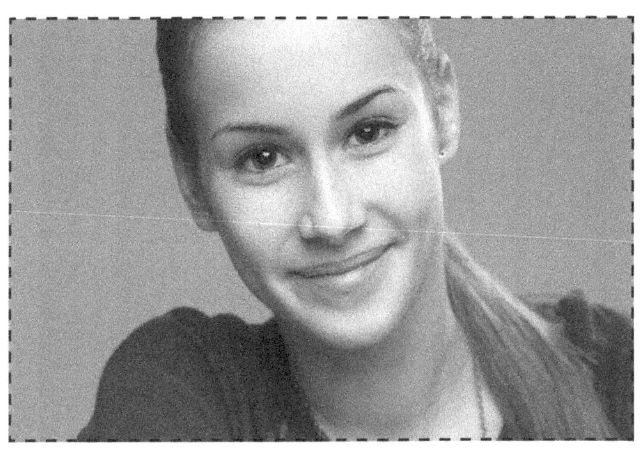
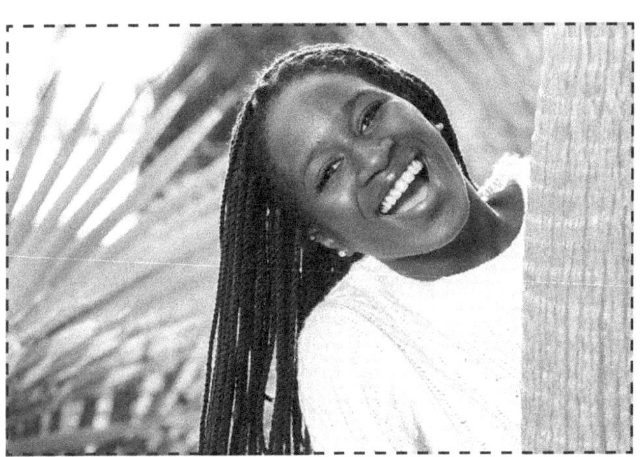
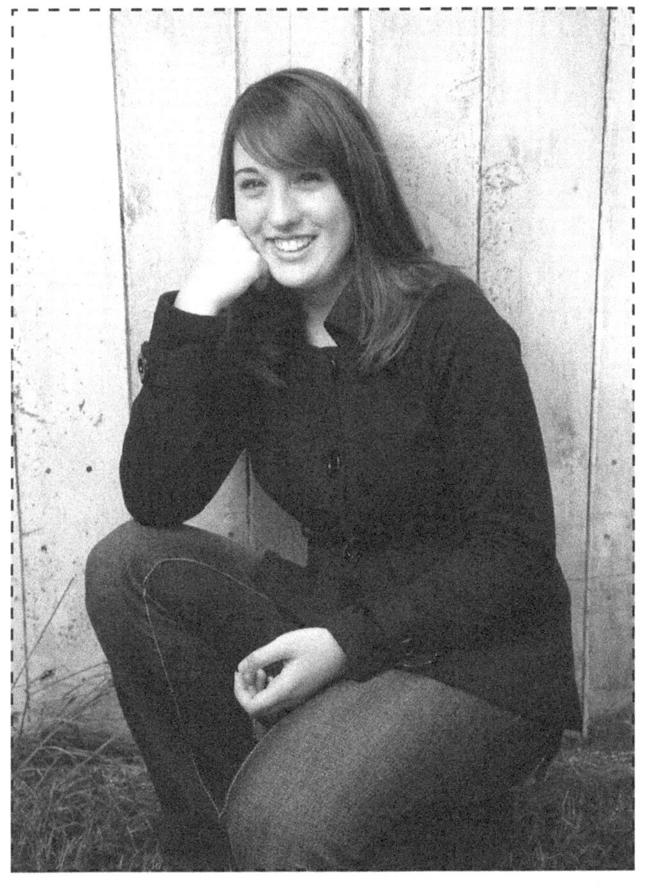
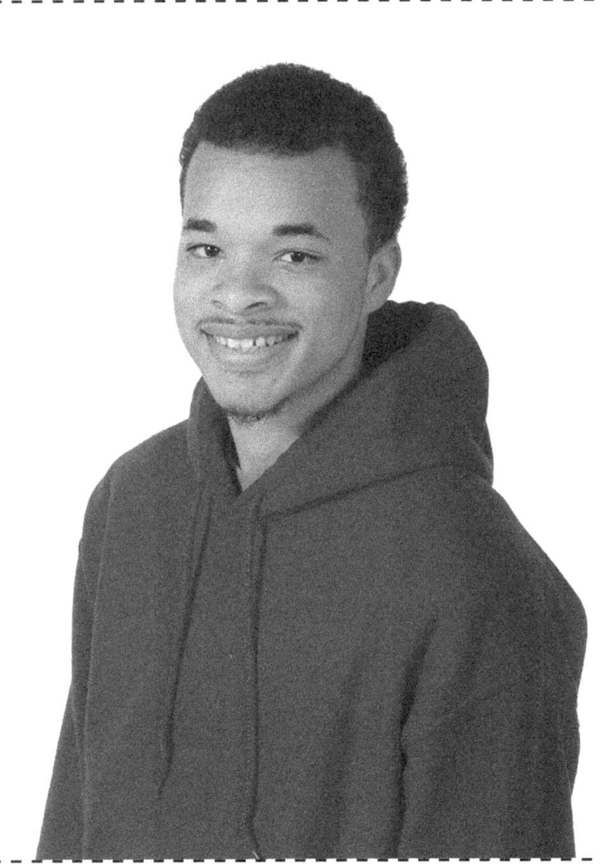

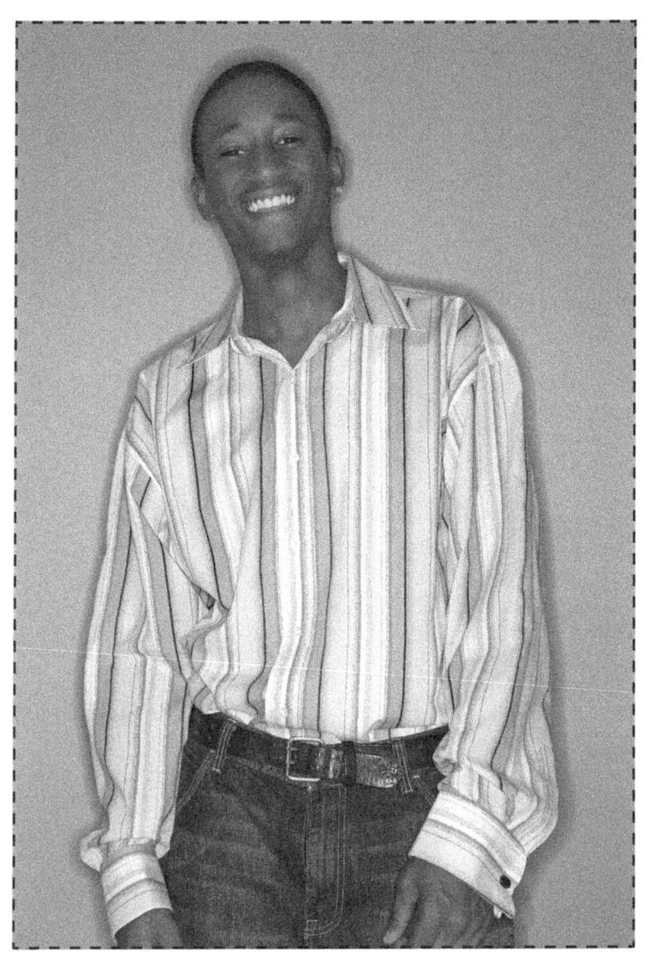

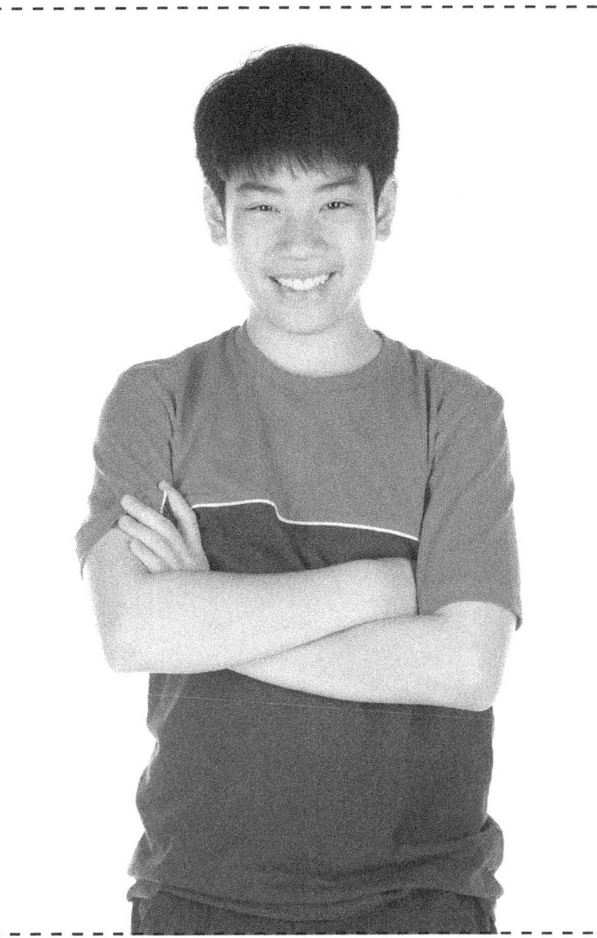

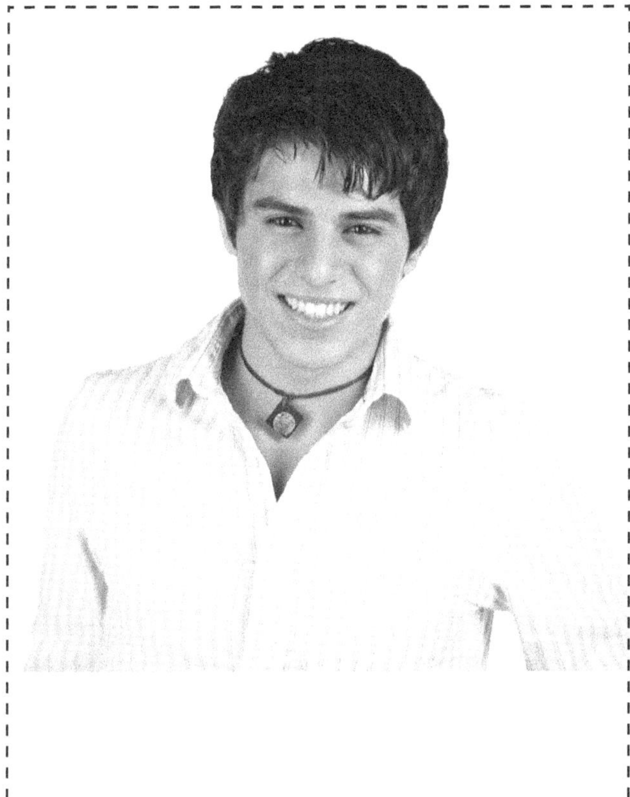

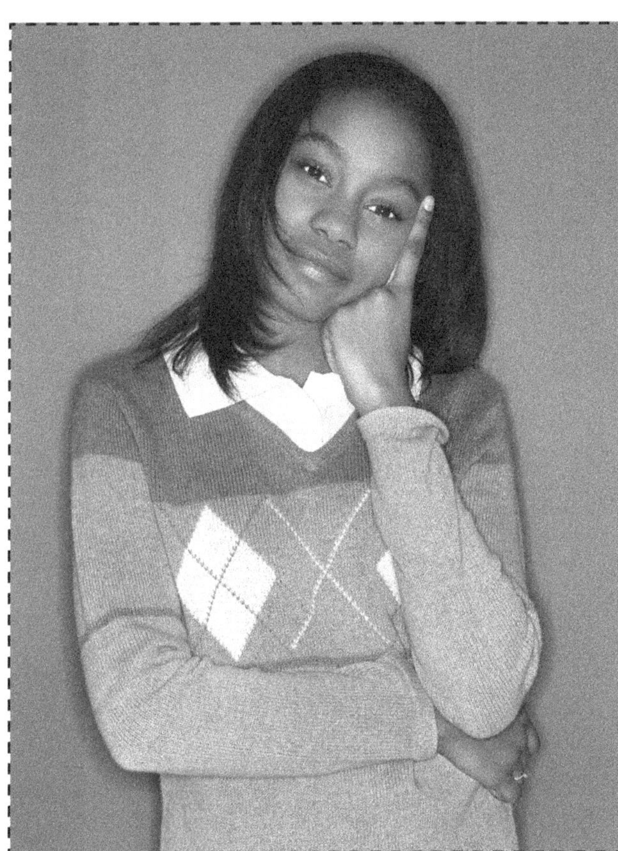

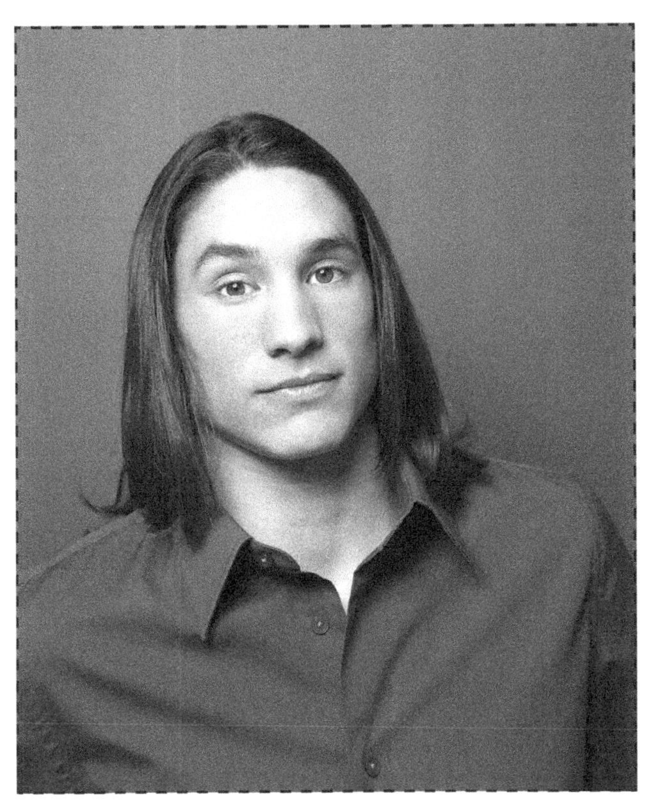

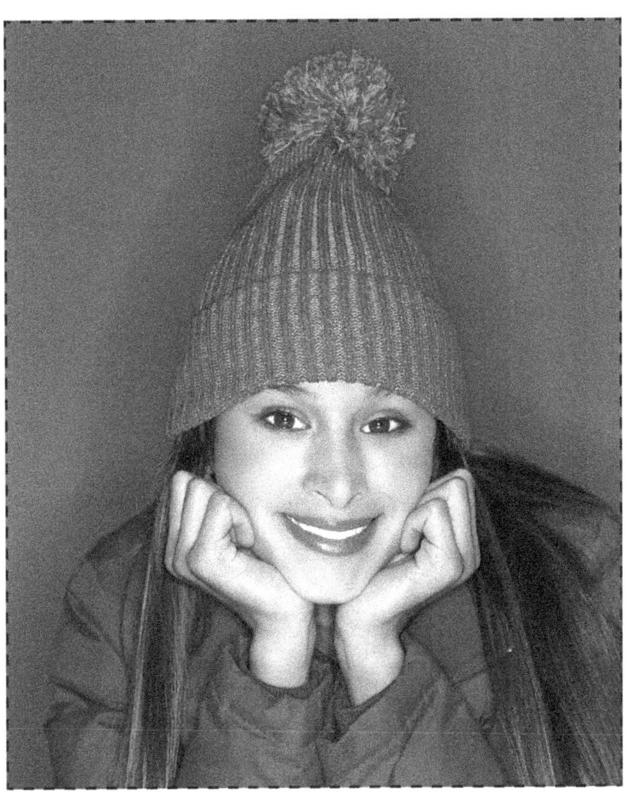

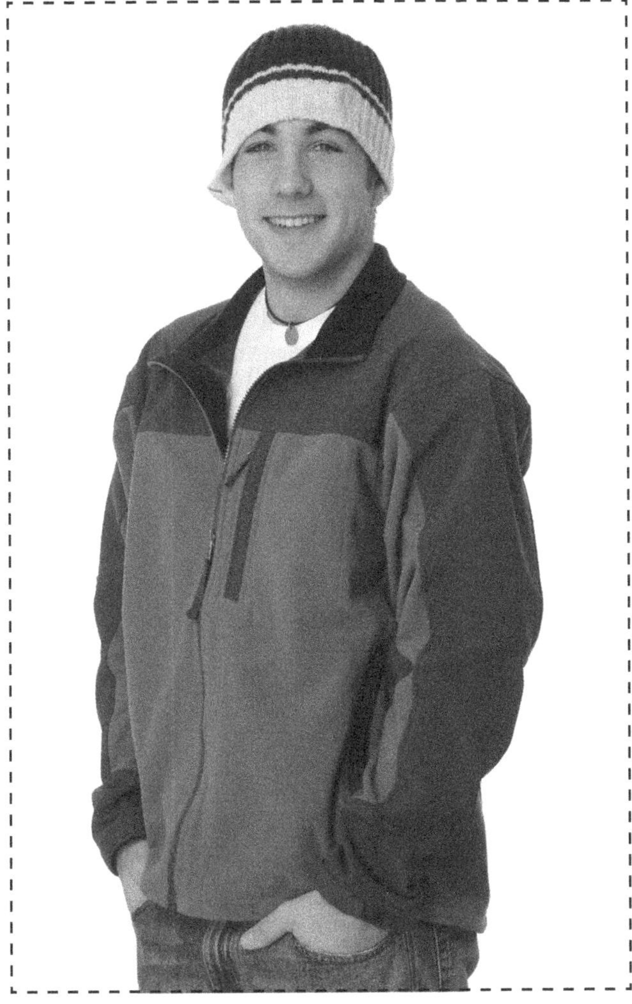

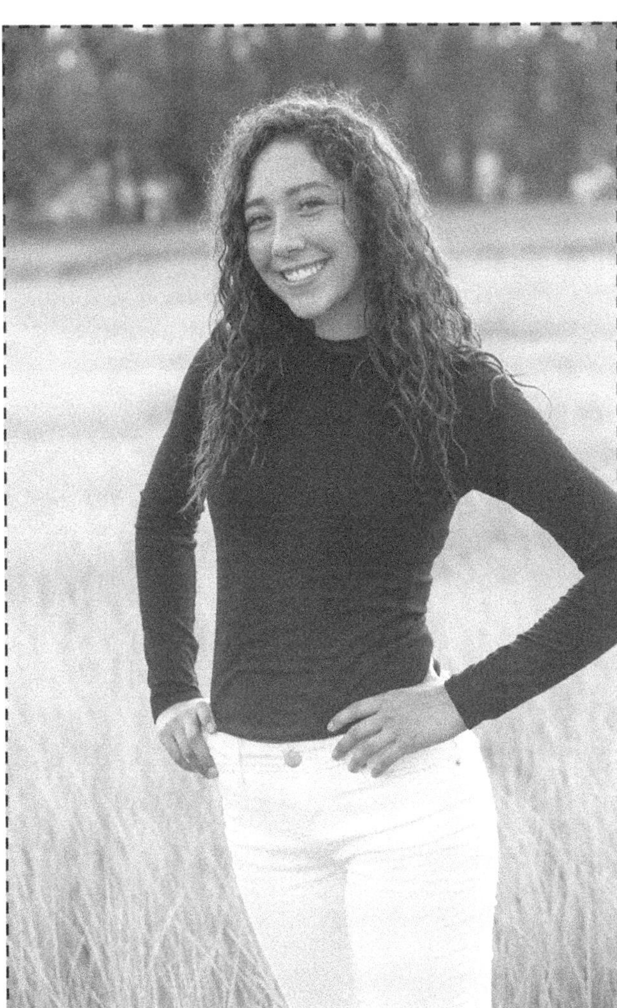

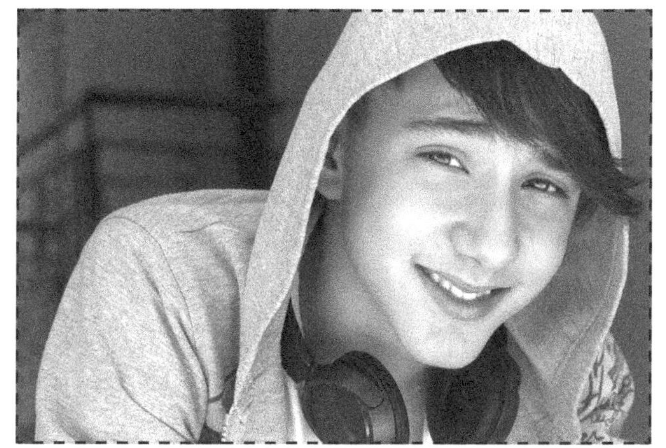

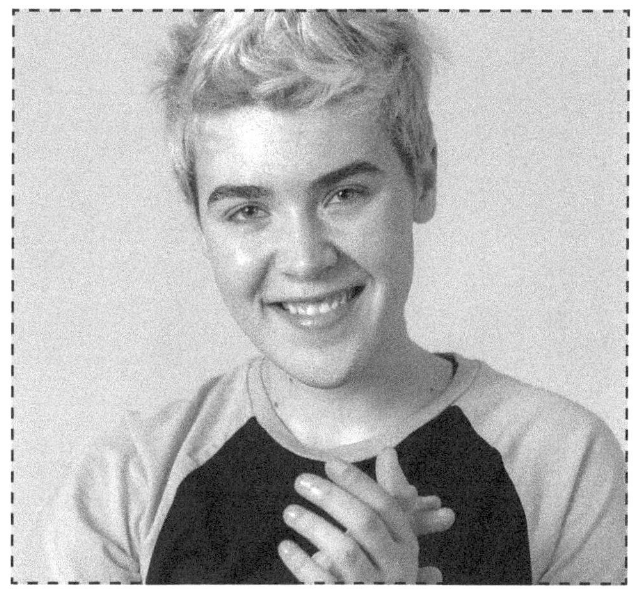

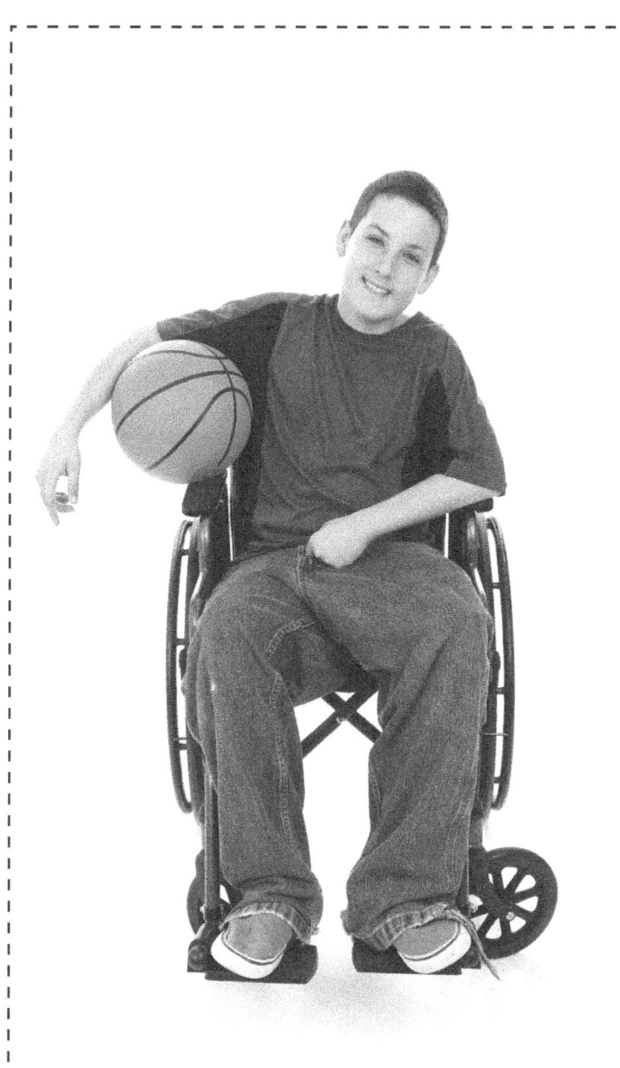

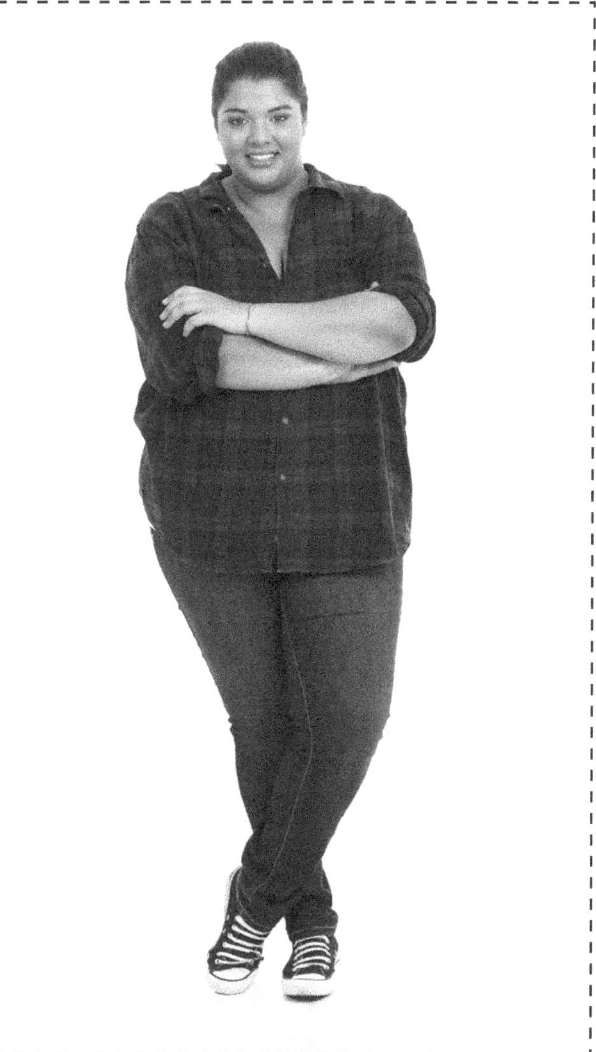

CONGRATULATIONS. THE CHILD/TEEN IS MORE PREPARED FOR VERBAL INTERACTIONS WITH OTHERS.

References

Abrahams, M. (2016). *Speaking up without freaking out*. Kendall Hunt Publishing.

Bergman, R. L., Keller, M. L., Piancentini, J., & Bergman, A. J. (2008). The development and psychometric properties of the Selective Mutism Questionnaire. *Journal of Child Clinical and Adolescent Psychology, 37*(2), 456–464.

Heinrich, P. (2018). *When role play comes alive: A theory and practice*. Springer Nature Singapore.

Kaplan, S. C., Morrison, A. S., Goldn, P. R., Olino, T. M., Heimberg, R. G., & Gross, J. J. (2017). The Cognitive Distortions Questionnaire (CD-Quest): Validation in a sample of adults with social anxiety disorder. *Cognitive Therapy and Research, 41*(4), 576–587.

APPENDIX A

DSM-5 DIAGNOSTIC CRITERIA FOR SELECTIVE MUTISM, CHILDHOOD-ONSET FLUENCY DISORDER (STUTTERING), AND SOCIAL (PRAGMATIC) COMMUNICATION DISORDER

The three disorders are separate diagnostic categories within the *Diagnostic and Statistical Manual of Mental Disorders, Fifth Edition* (*DSM-5*; American Psychiatric Association [APA], 2013). The ECHO Program addresses all three.

Selective Mutism falls within the Anxiety Disorders classification of the *DSM-5* (APA, 2013). These disorders are exemplified by excessive fear and anxiety related to behavioral disturbances with anticipation of future threat. Selective mutism may be diagnosed when the following criteria are met:

- There is a consistent failure to speak in specific social situations in which there is an expectation for speaking, such as at school, despite speaking in other situations.
- The failure to speak interferes with educational or occupational achievement or with social communication.
- The duration of the selective mutism is present for at least 1 month (not limited to the first month of school).
- The failure to speak is not due to lacking knowledge of, or comfort with, the spoken language required in the social situation.
- The disturbance is not better explained by a communication disorder (such as a childhood fluency disorder), schizophrenia, or another psychotic disorder.

According to the *DSM-5* (APA, 2013), *Childhood-Onset Fluency Disorder (Stuttering)* may be diagnosed when the following criteria are met:

- There is a disturbance in normal fluency and time patterning of speech inappropriate for the individual's age and skills with language that persists over time, characterized by one or more of the following:
  - ☐ sound and syllable repetitions
  - ☐ sound prolongations of consonants as well as vowels
  - ☐ broken words or pauses within a word
  - ☐ audible or silent blocking
  - ☐ circumlocutions

- ☐ words produced with excess physical tension
- ☐ monosyllabic whole-word repetitions

- The disturbance causes anxiety about speaking or limitations in effective communication, social participation, or academic or occupational performance.
- Onset of symptoms is early in development.
- The disturbance is not attributable to a sensory deficit, speech-motor deficit, associated neurological insult, or another medical condition and not better explained by another mental disorder.

According to the *DSM-5* (APA, 2013), *Social (Pragmatic) Communication Disorder* may be diagnosed when the following criteria are met:

- Persistent difficulties using verbal and nonverbal communication socially which may be manifested by the following four deficits:
  - ☐ using communication for social purposes appropriate for the social context, such as sharing information and engaging in greetings
  - ☐ changing communication to match the context or needs of the listener(s) for speaking differently to different people and in different situations
  - ☐ following rules of conversation and storytelling with turn-taking, rephrasing, and regulating interactions
  - ☐ understanding that which is not explicitly stated, such as inferences and interpretations based on context, idioms, and multiple meanings, to name a few
- The difficulties result in limitations of effective communication, social participation, social relationships, and academic or occupational performance.
- The symptoms begin in early development but may not become apparent until the demands of social communication exceed the child's capacities.
- The symptoms are not due to a medical or neurological condition or to low abilities in grammar, autism, intellectual disability, a mental disorder, or global developmental delay.

APPENDIX B

THE ECHO CHECKLIST

The ECHO Checklist is designed to gather information about the communication needs of children and teens with selective mutism or stuttering or others who can benefit from social pragmatic language practice.

The ECHO Checklist			
Directions: Read each item and check either YES or NO, and only select NOT SURE if you have no experience with the task. If you can do the task in one or two of the settings (home, school, or public places outside of school), underline the settings where you can do the task and do not underline the one that is difficult.			
	YES	**NO**	**NOT SURE**
1. I take turns listening and speaking in various settings (***at home, at school,*** and ***in public***).			
2. I give my conversation partner (another person) turns to talk too (***at home, at school,*** and ***in public***).			
3. I am aware of and speak about topics that interest the other person (***at home, at school,*** and ***in public***)			
4. I pay attention when the other person is talking (***at home, at school,*** and ***in public***).			
5. I keep a conversation going for a few minutes (***at home, at school,*** and ***in public***).			
6. I gesture with my hands at times when I speak (***at home, at school,*** and ***in public***).			
7. I speak so that the other person can hear what I say (***at home, at school,*** and ***in public***).			
8. I smile at times during a conversation (***at home, at school,*** and ***in public***).			
9. I nod to show I am listening when someone else is talking (***at home, at school,*** and ***in public***).			
10. I ask questions to show that I am interested in what someone says (***at home, at school,*** and ***in public***).			

continues

APPENDIX B. *continued*

	YES	NO	NOT SURE
11. I answer questions orally when someone asks me something (at home, at school, and ***in public***).			
12. I make comments that are related to someone's topic (***at home, at school,*** and ***in public***).			
13. I keep my body at an appropriate distance and posture when talking (***at home, at school,*** and ***in public***).			
14. I pause after some speaking to give someone time to think about what I said or to talk (***at home, at school,*** and ***in public***).			
15. I use eye contact to glance at and attend to someone who is talking (***at home, at school,*** and ***in public***).			
16. I speak with ease without feeling tightness in my throat in various situations (***at home, at school,*** and ***in public***)			
17. I use expression in my voice (variations in inflection/pitch) when I speak (***at home, at school,*** and ***in public***).			
18. I say hello or goodbye when entering or leaving (***at home, at school,*** and ***in public***).			
19. I don't hesitate to be the first to speak to other people (***at home, at school,*** and ***in public***).			
20. I say what I want and ask for what I need (***at home, at school,*** and ***in public***).			

ECHO PROGRAM—INFORMATION ABOUT ME

ECHO Program—Information About Me Name ____________________________ Date______________
Complete this information sheet as an interview or ask the person to write their answers.
1. My favorite hobbies and interests
2. The activities I like to do in or out of school
3. My favorite TV shows and movies
4. My favorite sites on the computer/Internet
5. Sports I enjoy watching or playing
6. My favorite music groups or artists
7. My favorite foods (snacks, meals, desserts)
8. My favorite things to do with electronic devices
9. Some of my favorite apps or websites
10. Pets at home and their ages and names
11. Favorite video games or board games
12. Anything else to share about my interests
13. What I like to do in my spare time
14. Interests I have that relate to a future job or career
15. Friends I like to spend time with

APPENDIX D

SOCIAL COMMUNICATION SKILLS—THE PRAGMATICS CHECKLIST

SOCIAL COMMUNICATION SKILLS—THE PRAGMATICS CHECKLIST				
Name ______________ Date ________ Completed by ____________ Relationship ____________ Read behaviors below and place an X in the column that best describes how words/language are used for each—**Pragmatic Objective**.	Not Present	Uses NO Words	Uses 1–3 Words	Uses Complex Language
INSTRUMENTAL—States needs				
1. Makes polite requests				
2. Makes choices				
3. Gives description of an object wanted				
4. Expresses a specific personal need				
5. Requests help				
REGULATORY—Gives commands/instructions				
6. Gives directions to play a game				
7. Gives directions to make something				
8. Changes style of commands/requests depending on who speaking to or what is wanted				
PERSONAL—Expresses feelings				
9. Identifies feelings (I'm happy.)				
10. Explains feelings (I'm happy because . . .)				
11. Provides excuses or reasons				
12. Offers an opinion with support				
13. Complains				
14. Blames others				

continues

APPENDIX D. *continued*

	Not Present	Uses NO Words	Uses 1–3 Words	Uses Complex Language
15. Provides pertinent information on request (2 or 3 for name, address, phone, birthdate)				
INTERACTIONAL—Me and You . . .				
16. Interacts with others in a polite manner				
17. Uses appropriate social rules such as greetings, farewells, thank you, getting attention				
18. Attends to the speaker				
19. Revises/repairs an incomplete message				
20. Initiates a topic of conversation				
21. Maintains a conversation (able to keep it going)				
22. Ends a conversation (doesn't just walk away)				
23. Interjects appropriately into an already established conversation with others				
24. Makes apologies or gives explanations of behavior				
25. Requests clarification				
26. States a problem				
27. Criticizes others				
28. Disagrees with others				
29. Compliments others				
30. Makes promises				
WANTS EXPLANATIONS—Tell me why . . .				
31. Asks questions to get more information				
32. Asks questions to systematically gather information as in "Twenty Questions"				
33. Asks questions because of curiosity				
34. Asks questions to problem solve (what should I do? How do I know?)				

	Not Present	Uses NO Words	Uses 1–3 Words	Uses Complex Language
35. Asks questions to make predictions (What will happen if . . . ?)				
SHARES KNOWLEDGE & IMAGINATIONS				
36. Role plays as/with different characters				
37. Role plays with props (one object used for another)				
38. Provides a description of a situation which describes the main events				
39. Correctly re-tells a story which has been told to them				
40. Relates the content of a 4-6 frame picture story using correct events for each frame				
41. Creates an original story with a beginning, several logical events, and an end				
42. Explains the relationship between two objects, actions or situation				
43. Compares and contrasts qualities of two objects, actions or situations				
44. Tells a lie				
45. Expresses humor/sarcasm				
TOTAL FOR EACH COLUMN				

Note. From "The Missing Link in Language Development: Social Communication Development," by D. Goberis, D. Beams, M. Dalpes, A. Abrisch, R. Baca, and C. Yoshinaga-Itano, 2012, *Seminars in Speech and Language, 33*(4), 297–309. Reprinted with permission © Georg Thieme Verlag KG.

APPENDIX E

EXPRESS SELECTIVE MUTISM (SM) COMMUNICATION QUESTIONNAIRE

Questionnaire begins on the following page.

Child's Name: ______________________ Today's Date: ______________

EXPRESS Selective Mutism (SM) Communication Questionnaire

Child's date of birth: ______________ Child's grade in school: ______________

Gender of child: Female _____ Male _____

Name of person completing form: ______________ Relationship: ______________

Language spoken at home by parents: ______________ and child: ______________

Is child bilingual: NO ____ or YES ____

Please indicate languages spoken fluently: ______________

Has your child received a formal diagnosis of selective mutism? YES ____ NO ____ NOT SURE ____

If yes, when diagnosed with SM (year) ______________ and by whom ______________

Diagnosis, Symptoms, and Treatment:

Has your child ever received any other diagnosis (listed below)? If treatment was provided, list dates. Indicate any symptoms you have observed. Check all that apply.

	Diagnosed (Year)	Received treatment	Even if no formal diagnosis, list symptoms observed
Development delay:	______	______	______
Speech-language impairment:	______	______	______
Sensory sensitivity:	______	______	______
Auditory processing issues:	______	______	______
Learning Disorder/Difference:	______	______	______
Anxiety Disorder:	______	______	______
Medical Conditions:	______	______	______
Attention Deficit Disorder:	______	______	______
Hyperactivity Disorder:	______	______	______
Other(s):	______	______	______

Questions about selective mutism:

When were you first made aware of your child's mutism? ______________ (age)

In what situation(s) was it noticed? ______________

____

Child's Name: ______________________________ **Today's Date:** ________________

Please describe your child's temperament/disposition around different people at home, in school, and in public places.

____

____

____

____

____

Is there a history of social anxiety, other anxiety problems, or phobias in the immediate or extended family? YES ____ NO ____

If yes, please explain:

____

____

____

____

In the box below, please describe what you might say or do to help your child communicate in various settings (at home, in school, and in public places).

Communication in various settings:

On next page: In the three settings listed on the chart below (home, school, and public places), please indicate how your child communicates with those listed. Write a sentence or two to describe the ways in which your child communicates with others. In situations where your child has had no opportunity to meet and interact with those people or situations listed below, write NA for "Not Applicable." Also, indicate if your child only responds or responds and initiates. Please note if child whispered, spoke in single words, used sentences, or engaged in spontaneous conversation. Also note if nonverbal using gestures or communicating by writing.

Child's Name: ______________________ Today's Date: ______________

WRITE IN BOXES	Home	School	Public
Immediate Family	At home with family, how does your child communicate? ____ responds /____ initiates	How does your child communicate with a family member at school? ____ responds /____ initiates	How does your child communicate with a family member when out in public? ____ responds /____ initiates
Relatives	When relatives visit the home, how does your child communicate with them? ____ responds /____ initiates	If a relative is at school, how does your child communicate with him/her? ____ responds /____ initiates	When your with a relative in public, how does your child communicate with him/her? ____ responds /____ initiates
Adult Friends of Family and Peers	When an adult friend visits the home, how does your child communicate with him/her? ____ responds /____ initiates	If an adult friend is at school, how does your child communicate with him/her? ____ responds /____ initiates	When in a public place with an adult friend, how does your child communicate? ____ responds /____ initiates
Neighbors	If neighbors visit the home, how does your child communicate with them? ____ responds /____ initiates	If a neighbor is at your child's school, how does your child communicate with him/her? ____ responds /____ initiates	If in a public place with a neighbor (and parent), how does your child communicate? ____ responds /____ initiates
Store Clerks	Not Applicable X	Not Applicable X	How does your child communicate with a store clerk? ____ responds /____ initiates

Child's Name: ______________________________ Today's Date: ________________

WRITE IN BOXES	Home	School	Public
Servers	Not Applicable X	Not Applicable X	How does your child communicate with a server at a restaurant? ____ responds/____ initiates
Doctors/ Helping Professionals	If a helping professional (such as a therapist or counselor, etc.) worked with your child at home, how did your child communicate? ____ responds/____ initiates	If a helping professional (such as nurse, counselor, etc.) is working with your child at school, how does your child communicate? ____ responds/____ initiates	How does your child communicate with a doctor or other helping professional at their office? ____ responds/____ initiates
Peers	When a peer visits the home, how does your child communicate with him/her? ____ responds/____ initiates	How does your child communicate with peers at school? Consider one peer, small group, and classroom. ____ responds/____ initiates	When in a public place with a peer (and a parent), how does your child communicate? How does your child communicate if playing at a peer's house? ____ responds/____ initiates
Teachers	If a teacher visits the home, how does your child communicate with him/her? ____ responds/____ initiates	How does your child communicate with teachers in school when alone with the teacher or in the group? ____ responds/____ initiates	If a teacher is seen in a public place, how does your child communicate with him/her? ____ responds/____ initiates
Others	____ responds/____ initiates	____ responds/____ initiates	____ responds/____ initiates

Child's Name: ______________________________ **Today's Date:** ________________

How does your child communicate in various settings when you are there compared to when you are not there? Please describe.

How does your child communicate on the phone with anyone who may call? Please describe.

How does your child like school? Please describe.

Has your child ever received any type of treatment/therapy/medication for selective mutism? If yes, please explain your child's progress and difficulties.

Child's Name: ______________________________ **Today's Date:** ________________

As best you can, please provide an overview of your child's selective mutism and any information you believe important to share. In doing so, please provide details of your child's social world and communication skills and difficulties. Include anything your child has told you about talking including what helps or what is difficult.

INDEX

Note: Page numbers in **bold** reference non-text material

B

C

D

E

S

T

U

V

W

Y